MANUAL OF DRY NEEDLING TECHNIC

Volume 1 (Upper & Lower Quarter)

FIRST EDITION

Foreword

It is my proud privilege to write foreward to this most needed book. Dry needling technique has come a long way since in the management of pain, trigger points & related syndromes. In a short span of time, it became successful to draw attention of many health care service providers across globe. In India, the number of patients getting benefits from this technique is increasing day by day. I was able to get relief from prolonged shin splint & fascia tightness because of this technique which Piyush Jain introduced to me three years back. Dry needling is gaining popularity in India & around globe. Despite this, there was relative lack of books which explains this technique in simpler language & also adequately supported with pictorial presentations of each muscle. Piyush Jain's effort to address this issue is quite appreciable.

He took effort to present this technique & shared his experience in the simplest manner. The method is explained in precise & concise manner. Besides the ample of diagrams & text, this book draws reader's attention towards trigger points pathology & anatomical correlations of muscles. Attempt has made to give explanation in relation with anatomy with diagram & also quadrants.

Piyush Jain has made use of his several years of experience & expertise to construct this practical guide. Written in clear & lucid style without getting bogged down in trivia that might put off most readers, it covers the basics of dry needling technique in refreshing readable manner. This book will be great information resource to students & clinicians who want to be self sufficient in application of this technique.

I would unhesitatingly recommend this book to all health care professionals who are associated with use of this technique for better care of their patients. I can confidently say that Piyush Jain's work would go long way in making a complex topic more amenable to those who seek better understanding of dry needling technique.

Dr. Sudeep Kale
Associate Professor,
Terna Physiotherapy College, Navi Mumbai
Ph.D Scholar,
Maharashtra University of Health Sciences, Nasik

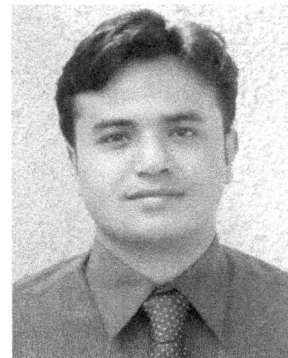

.

Foreword

"Wow! It's so amazing!" These were my words after reading the manuscript of this book. I know Piyush Jain since many years and his passion for his work always motivates me. I had read his last book – "Manual of Kinesiological Taping: An Epitome of Kinesiology Taping Techniques" and that time I realized that he has something different in his writing skill. The way he formulates the sentences and uses the pictures/ diagrams, it gives an experience of learning in the class.

Since 1942 when Dr. Travell proposed injections into MTrPs, lot of things has been changed. Though Karel Lewit had already proposed in 1979 that the effect of injections were actually the effect of needling, the research of Dr. Chang Hong in 1994 brought a new revolution in the field of myofascial pain management. And now Dr. Travell's idea of injection has turned into the idea of dry needling... a current trend worldwide.

This book is a self-study course in itself. Where the text on the physiological aspects and discussion on the different models make it useful for the DN practitioners, the inclusion of even the basic and minor details in each chapter makes it easier for the students to learn. This book not only exposes the readers to the basic levels but also constrains them to push themselves to the peak of the Bloom's Taxonomy.

I am happy to share that I have already listed this book as a recommended book in the syllabus of St. Louis University, Cameroon (West-Central Africa). I would like to recommend this book to all the health professionals who want to learn DN.

Happy Learning!

Dr. Krishna N. Sharma
Dean
 HOD (Physiotherapy) - St. Louis University, Cameroon
Author of more than 100 books & 2 Bestsellers
3 Times World Record Holder
www.drkrishna.co.in

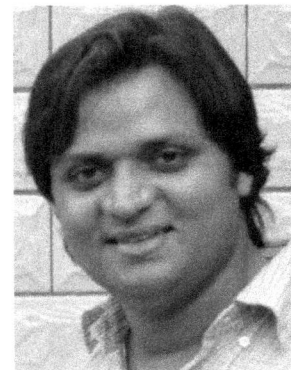

Dedications:

This book is dedicated to:

My idol Joginder Yadav sir

My parents Aruna Jain and Ramesh Chand Jain

My brothers Ayush Jain and Mayank Jain

To my better half Dr. Tanvi Jain.

Acknowledgement

A special thanks to Dr. Krishna N. Sharma and Dr. Sudeep Kale for being an inspiration for me to write this text, and helping me in all the stages required to complete this book.

I would like to thank my big brother Dr. Joji. M. John, whose critical analyses of the text and of the author, made me strong and motivated towards completing the book to best of its quality. The courtesy for trigger point illustrations goes to my friend Dr. Vishal Goel who worked many days to draw these and our model Deepak.

I would like to thank special professionals who helped not only in this book but in every stage of life, Thanks Dr. Umasankar Mohanty, Dr. Manish Arora, Dr. Anand Mishra, Dr. Ketan Bhatikar, Dr. Sanjiv Jha, Dr. Einstein Jerome, Dr. Sanjay Parmar, Dr. Anjani Kumar, Dr. Gaurish Kenkre, Dr. Mihir Somaiya and all my friends, colleagues and professionals.

MANUAL OF DRY NEEDLING TECHNIQUES

Volume 1 (Upper & Lower Quarter)

FIRST EDITION

PIYUSH JAIN

B.P.T, M.P.T (Ortho), CKTT (Germany), CCN, CSN, CDCO, MIAP, MIAMSE (West Virginia, USA), MISEI.

Founder: Institute Of Kinesiology Taping.

President: Physical Therapy Research and Education Foundation.

PREF PUBLICATIONS

(INDIA)

PUBLISHED BY:

PREF
PUBLICATIONS

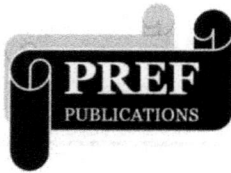

PREF PUBLICATIONS, INDIA

Copyright © 2015 by PIYUSH JAIN

Contact details (for permission): piyush_2506@yahoo.co.in, 9868418040

First Edition, 2015

Published in Delhi, India

ISBN- 978-81-924267-2-3

Notice:

Neither the publisher nor the author assume any responsibility for any loss, injury or damage to person or property arising out of use of content of this book. It is the responsibility of the therapist, to determine the best application of techniques to the patients.

The publisher

Printed by:
Creative Digital Publication Pvt. Ltd.
Mob. 09891609549

PREFACE

Dry Needling methods can help in providing the healthcare professionals a great tool to serve their patients with great result in conjunction to other therapeutic modalities. No treatment protocol can work without a proper assessment of the patients, the need of clinical reasoning with proper assessment tools are the basic necessity of the therapist. In 1942 Dr. Travell proposed injections into MTrPs, though in 1979 Karel Lewit proposed the effect of injections were actually the effect of needling since then the use of Dry needling technique came into picture. And now Dr. Travell's idea of injection has turned into the idea of dry needling and many researches came up with it efficacy and reliability. As it became famous the confusion about it as being part of acupuncture also gains popularity. The only thing in dry needing which has a bit of acupuncture in it, are the needles which is being used by the therapist.

As Per American Academy of Orthopedic Manual Physical Therapists (AAOMPT)
"Dry needling is a neurophysiological evidence-based treatment technique that requires effective manual assessment of the neuromuscular system. Physical therapists are well trained to utilize dry needling in conjunction with manual physical therapy interventions. Research supports that dry needling improves pain control, reduces muscle tension, normalizes biochemical and electrical dysfunction of motor endplates, and facilitates an accelerated return to active rehabilitation."

The statement above is self explanatory on the functional, physiological and medical aspect of treatment. This book is a basic reference text for the therapists who are trained in the method of dry needling procedures in accordance to norm of practice of their respective countries. The basic steps given in the book can make a practicing therapist to use dry needling technique for the subjects in different clinical conditions. The text focus not only on the steps needed to be performed but also focus on what should not be done by a therapist while performing the procedure. At work we have taken all the guidelines given by OSHA for blood borne diseases as well as WHO guideline on workplace and hand hygiene.

As dry needling is an emerging field in India, there is great need of good therapists and researchers in this field. The book's content may be revised time to time with latest advancements, new researches and human errors if any.

PIYUSH JAIN
PHYSIOTHERAPIST
INDIA

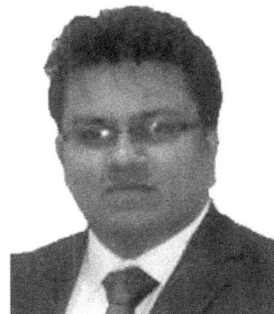

Contents

CHAPTER 1 - INTRODUCTION

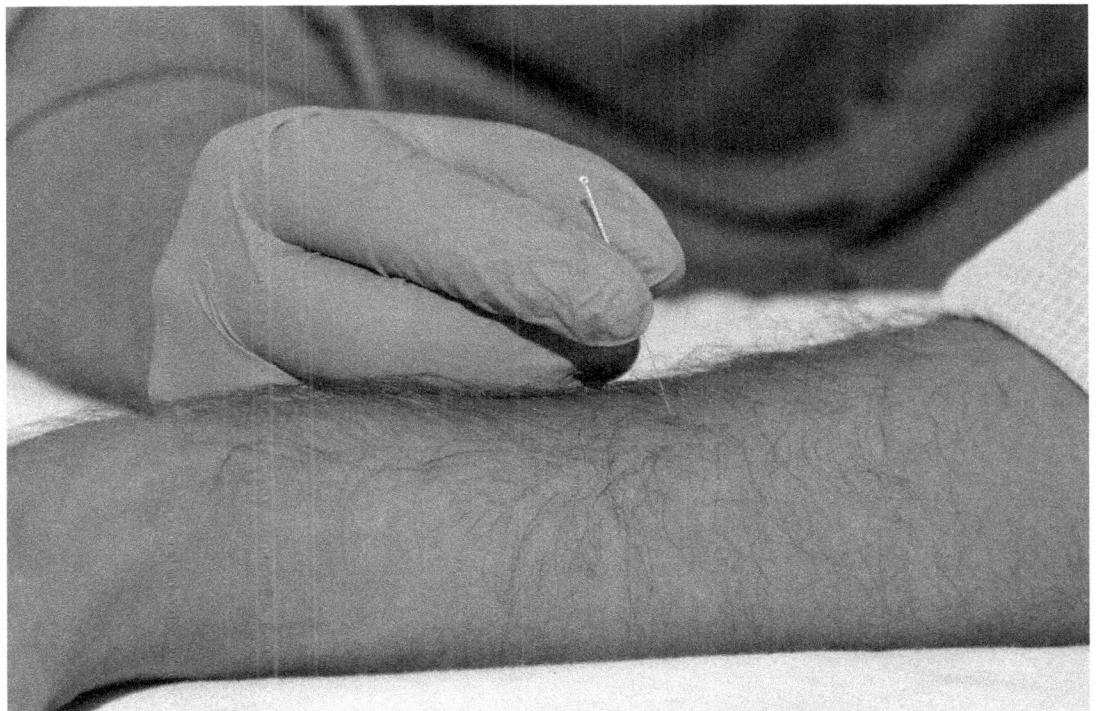

Introduction

History

In 1979, Dr. Karel Lewit reported his stunning success with a large number of patients with musculoskeletal pain by employing nothing more than what is described as "dry needling." Dry needling refers to the therapeutic effect of applying needle stimulation directly to trigger points without the use of injection. Dry needling utilizes a solid filament needle, as is used in the practice of acupuncture, but its gauge varies depending on the area of treatment. It mechanically disrupts the integrity of the dysfunctional endplates within the trigger area, resulting in mechanical and physiological resolution of the TrPs. It also shows a strong pain-inhibitory role by opioids released through needle stimulation of A-delta receptors. The approach of dry needling is based on Western anatomical and neurophysiological principles. This should not to be confused with the traditional Chinese medicine (TCM) rationale for the stimulation of acupuncture points. Lewit, in 1979 published one of the first review in the medical literature. He reported that dry needling of myofascial trigger points caused immediate analgesia at almost 87% of the needle sites, which he referred to as the "needle effect." Nearly a third of subjects remained free of pain. About 20% of subjects experienced several months without pain, 22% several weeks, 11% several days, and approximately 14% had no pain relief. Lewit observed that the effectiveness of dry needling was directly related to the accuracy of needling , which depends greatly on the ability to palpate myofascial trigger points accurately. In 1980, Gunn et al. published a prospective dry needling study of injured workers with low back pain and demonstrated that dry needling was an effective treatment for low back pain. Dr. Chan Gunn, M.D., is the founder of dry needling in Canada. He wrote "As a first step toward acceptance of acupuncture by the medical profession, it is suggested that a new system of acupuncture locus nomenclature be introduced, relating them to known neural structures." One may reasonably infer from this statement that Dr, Gunn believed that in order for acupuncture to be accepted in Western medicine, the technique would need to be redefined.

There are similarities, but also very significant differences between the TCM style of acupuncture and dry needling. Acupuncture follows rules and beliefs that have been established since ancient times, whereas dry needling ignores ancient acupuncture philosophy. Most, if not all of TCM, is based on pre-scientific ideas, whereas dry needling is totally based on modern scientific neurophysiology and anatomy. Dry needling is purely for pain relief and based on recent understandings in pain science. There is much less mystique surrounding dry needling for pain abatement. TCM acupuncture can treat a vast range of somato viscero illnesses, as well as being effective in pain relief. In contrast, dry needling is specifically used for pain control of the musculoskeletal system. Therefore, acupuncture will always be a viable treatment option for both internal disorders as well as musculoskeletal involvements.

In the evaluation of pain, there are two primary types: neuropathic pain from a damaged or dysfunctional nerve, and nociceptive pain, which is very common, caused by osteoarthritis, headaches, sprains/strains, myofascial pain, etc. Both of these pain types have shown extremely good response to dry needling of associated trigger points.

Whereas the origin of the term "Dry Needling" is attributed to Janet G. Travell, M.D. In her book, 'Myofascial Pain and Dysfunction: Trigger Point Manual', Dr. Travell uses the term "dry needling" to differentiate between two hypodermic needle techniques when performing trigger point therapy. The two techniques she described are the injection of a local anesthetic and the mechanical use of a hypodermic needle without injecting a solution (Travell, Simons, & Simons, 1999, pp. 154–155). Dr. Travell preferred a 22-gauge, 1.5-in hypodermic needle for trigger point therapy and used this needle for both injection therapy and dry needling. Dr. Travell had access to acupuncture needles but reasoned that they were far too thin for trigger point therapy. She preferred hypodermic needles because of their strength and tactile feedback:"A 22-gauge, 3.8-cm (1.5-in) needle is usually suitable for most superficial muscles. In hyperalgesic patients a 25-gauge, 3.8-cm (1.5-in) needle may cause less discomfort, but will not provide the clear "feel" of the structures being penetrated by needle and is more likely to be deflected by the dense contraction knots that are the target. A 27-gauge needle, 3.8-cm (1.5-in) needle is even more flexible; the tip is more likely to be deflected by the contraction knots and it provides less tactile feedback for precision injection" (Travell, Simons, & Simons, 1999, p. 156).

The use of a hypodermic needle for dry needling was described by Dr. Chang-Zern Hong in his research paper on "Lidocaine Injection Verses Dry Needling to Myofascial Trigger Point". In his research, he describes the procedure for trigger point injection and dry needling by using a 27-gauge hypodermic needle 1 ¼-in long (Hong, 1994). Both Travell and Hong used hypodermic needles for dry needling. Dr. Hong, unlike Dr. Travell, did not use an acupuncture needle for dry needling.

Although dry needling originally utilized only hypodermic needles due to the concern that solid filiform needles had neither the strength or tactile feedback that hypodermic needles provided and that the solid filiform needle could be deflected by "dense contraction knots", those concerns have proven false and many healthcare practitioners who perform dry needling have found that the solid filiform needles not only provides better tactile feedback but also penetrate the "dense muscle knots" better and are easier to manage and caused less discomfort to patients. For that reason both the use of hypodermic needles and the use of solid filiform needles are now accepted in dry needling practice.

Dry needling using solid filiform needles contrasts with the use of a hollow hypodermic needle used to inject substances such as saline solution, botox or corticosteroids to the same point. Such use of a solid needle has been found to be as effective as injection of substances in such cases as relief of pain in muscles and connective tissue. Analgesia produced by needling a pain spot has been called the needle effect.

Dry needling is quickly becoming a very popular modality in healthcare profession internationally, as musculoskeletal complaints are one of the most reported conditions for which people seek professional attention. By deactivating TrPs using needle stimulation directly into the trigger point, the reported pain relief is noteworthy. It does not require background on the theoretical foundations of Chinese medicine, nor does it deal with the myriad of ancient laws surrounding the practice of acupuncture. It is quick, easy and very effective. In acupuncture, it may sometimes be referred to as "surrounding the dragon," which simply implies stimulating painful points in and around the area of the involvement. My personal evaluation of this approach of needling for musculoskeletal pain is that it is directly related to the musculo-tendino meridian, as opposed to the primary meridians of the body.

Dry needling is based entirely on the neurophysiologically modern understanding of pain as it surrounds hyperactive trigger points in a specific area. The diagnosis is totally based upon palpation. Contracted muscle fibers provide resistance to the needle and may cause a "needle grasp." This phenomenon causes a deep ache, which in acupuncture is described as de qi.

In essence, both acupuncture and dry needling make use of the needle as their primary modality. Trigger points likewise can be influenced by high-impact percussion over the area, which is noninvasive but may have less response than needle stimulation.

Around the world, physicians of all disciplines are utilizing dry needling over trigger points, with outstanding clinical success. Its growth as a medically accepted therapy is preceded only by the growth of acupuncture in North America. Even though there are similarities between acupuncture and dry needling, the primary difference is the rationale on how the condition is approached. It is an internationally accepted, scientific, neurophysiologic treatment approach that is gaining wide popularity as its use by the health care professions accelerates.

Dry needling for the treatment of myofascial (muscular) trigger points is based on theories similar, but not exclusive, to traditional acupuncture: however, dry needling targets the trigger points, which is the direct and palpable source of patient pain, rather than the traditional "meridians", accessed via acupuncture. The distinction between trigger points and acupuncture points for the relief of pain is blurred. As reported by Melzack, et al., there is a high degree of correspondence (71% based on their analysis) between published locations of trigger points and classical acupuncture points for the relief of pain. What distinguishes dry needling from traditional acupuncture is that it does not use the full range of traditional theories of Chinese Medicine. The debated distinction between dry needling and acupuncture has become a controversy because it relates to an issue of scope of practice of various professions.

International Definitions of Dry Needling

- As per February 2013 APTA version of this document titled, Description of Dry Needling in Clinical Practice: an Educational Resource Paper, defines dry needling as:
  "Dry needling is a skilled intervention that uses a thin filiform needle to penetrate the skin and stimulate underlying myofascial trigger points, muscular, and connective tissues for the management of neuromusculoskeletal pain and movement impairments"

- As per the statement given by American Academy of Orthopedic Manual Physical Therapists (AAOMPT) **"Dry needling is a neurophysiological evidence-based treatment technique that requires effective manual assessment of the neuromuscular system. Physical therapists are well trained to utilize dry needling in conjunction with manual physical therapy interventions. Research supports that dry needling improves pain control, reduces muscle tension, normalizes biochemical and electrical dysfunction of motor endplates, and facilitates an accelerated return to active rehabilitation."**

- The Mississippi State Board of Physical Therapy define it as **"Intramuscular manual therapy is a physical intervention that uses a filiform needle no larger than a 25-gauge needle to stimulate trigger points, diagnose and treat neuromuscular pain and functional movement deficits; is based upon Western medical concepts; requires an examination and diagnosis, and treats specific anatomic entities selected according to physical signs".**

- Irish Society of Charted Physiotherapist mentioned in a draft as **" Dry Needling (DN) is a term referring to the employment of a solid filament needle for the treatment of pain and / or dysfunction of various body tissues. DN is considered an invasive physical therapy technique. There are a variety of conceptual models, most commonly DN is employed to treat myofascia including myofascial trigger points (TrPs)(Travell and Simons 1983; Travell and Simons 1992; Simons, Travell et al. 1999). The term Trigger Point Dry Needling (TrPDN) refers to the treatment of TrPs with dry needling techniques.**

Dry needling is a skilled intervention used by physical therapists that uses a thin filiform needle to penetrate the skin and stimulate underlying myofascial trigger points, muscular, and connective tissues for the management of neuromusculoskeletal pain and movement impairments. A trigger point describes a taut band of skeletal muscle located within a larger muscle group. Trigger points can be tender to the touch and can refer pain to distant parts of the body. Physical therapists utilize dry needling with the goal of releasing/inactivating the trigger points and relieving pain. Preliminary research supports that dry needling improves pain control, reduces muscle tension, normalizes biochemical and electrical dysfunction of motor endplates, and facilitates an accelerated return to active rehabilitation.

The physiological basis for DN depends upon the targeted tissue and treatment objectives. The treatment of myofascial trigger points (referred to as TrPs) has a different physiological basis than treatment of excessive muscle tension, scar tissue, fascia, and connective tissues. TrPs are hyperirritable spots within a taut band of skeletal muscle fibers that produce local and/or referred pain when stimulated. TrPs are divided into active and latent TrPs dependent upon the degree of irritability. Active TrPs are spontaneously painful, while latent TrPs are only painful when stimulated, for example, with digital pressure. TrPs can be visualized by magnetic resonance imaging and sonography elastography, which has shown that active TrPs are larger than latent TrPs and feature a reduction in circulation. TrPs are physiological contractures, characterized by local ischemia and hypoxia, a significantly lowered pH (active TRPs only), a chemically altered milieu (active TRPs only), local and referred pain, and altered muscle activation patterns. Although latent TrPs are not spontaneously painful, recent research has shown that they do contribute to nociception, therefore they need to be included in the treatment plan. TrPs are associated with dysfunctional motor endplates, endplate noise, and an increased release of acetylcholine. TrPs activate muscle nociceptors and are peripheral sources of persistent nociceptive input, thus contributing to the development of peripheral and central sensitization. Stimulation of TrPs activates the periaqueductal grey and anterior cingular cortex in the brain, and enkaphalinergic, serotonergic, and noradrenergic inhibitory systems associated with A-δ (A delta) fibers through segmental inhibition.

DN can be divided into deep and superficial DN. Deep DN has been shown to inactivate TrPs by eliciting local twitch responses (LTR), which are modulated by the central nervous system. A LTR is a spinal cord reflex that is characterized by an involuntary contraction of the contractured taut band,which can be elicited by a snapping palpation or penetration with a needle. The LTR has been shown to be associated with alleviation and mitigation of spontaneous electrical activity or motor endplate noise; a reduction of the concentration of numerous nociceptive, inflammatory, and immune system related chemicals and relaxation of the taut band. Deep DN of TrPs is associated with reduced local and referred pain, improved range of motion, and decreased TrP irritability both locally and more remotely. DN normalizes the chemical milieu and pH of skeletal muscle and restores the local circulation. Superficial DN is thought to activate mechanoreceptors coupled to slow conducting unmyelinated C fiber afferents, and indirectly, stimulate the anterior cingular cortex. Superficial DN may also be mediated through stimulation of A-δ fibers, or via stretching of fibroblasts in connective tissue. Superficial DN is associated with reduced local and referred pain and improved range of motion, but it is not known at this time whether superficial DN has any impact on normalizing the chemical environment of active TrPs or reducing motor endplate noise associated with TrPs in general.

The physiological basis for DN treatment of excessive muscle tension, scar tissue, fascia, and connective tissues is not as well described in the literature, but the available research shows that there may be several benefits. Muscle tension is determined by a combination of the basic viscoelastic properties of a muscle and its surrounding fascia, and the degree of activation of the contractile apparatus of the muscle. There is some evidence that excessive muscle tension, as seen for example in spasticity, can be alleviated with DN. Scar tissue has been linked to myofascial pain and fibroblasts. Fibroblasts are specialized contractile cells within the fascia that are of particular interest, as they synthesize, organize, and remodel collagen, dependent upon the tension between the extracellular matrix and the cell. DN, especially when used in combination with rotation of the needle, can place fibroblasts in a high tension matrix, at which point the fibroblast changes shape and assumes a lamellar shape, and increases its collagen synthesis and cell proliferation. DN has been shown to directly activate fibroblasts through mechanical manipulation of the needle, which in turn activates the release of cytokines and other pro-inflammatory mediators. DN can play a substantial role in the process of mechano transduction, which is described as the process by which the body converts mechanical loading into cellular responses. Fibroblast activation with a solid filament has been shown to result in pain neuromodulation.

Indications for Use

DN may be incorporated into a treatment plan when myofascial TrPs are present, which may lead to impairments in body structure, pain, and functional limitations. TrPs are sources of persistent peripheral nociceptive input and their inactivation is consistent with current pain management insights. DN also is indicated with restrictions in range of motion due to contracture muscle fibers or taut bands, or other soft tissue restrictions, such as fascial adhesions or scar tissue. TrPs have been identified in numerous diagnoses, such as radiculopathies, joint dysfunction, disk pathology, tendonitis, craniomandibular dysfunction, migraines, tension-type headaches, carpal tunnel syndrome, computer-related disorders, whiplash associated disorders, spinal dysfunction,pelvic pain and other urologic syndromes, post-herpetic neuralgia, complex regional pain syndrome, nocturnal cramps, phantom pain, and other relatively uncommon diagnoses such as Barré Liéou syndrome, or neurogenic pruritus, among others.

Further in the chapter we will be discussing about the pain pathways, basics of trigger points and deep dry needling techniques of upper and lower quarter muscles in details. Before starting the procedure we will be giving very brief details about the basics of pain and pain modulation.

Introduction to pain

Pain is a sub modality of somatic sensation. The word "pain" is described as a broad range of unpleasing sensory and emotional experiences presented with genuine or possible tissue damage. Pain is a signal that we cannot ignore. Pain sensation is carried to the CNS via three major pathways. The ability to diagnose diseases depends on the specific knowledge of the multiple qualities and factors related to pain. Sensitivity and reaction to noxious stimuli are essential for the well-being and survival of an individual. Pain travels via redundant pathways, ensures to inform the individual: "Get out of this situation immediately." Without these attributes, the individual has no means of preventing or minimizing tissue injury. Individuals congenitally possessing insensitivity to pain are easily injured and usually die at an early age.

For many years, physicians tried to manage pain without the details in which pain is indicated from the injured part to the brain. Recent findings about how the body notices, carries and responds to painful stimuli, have allowed professionals to relieve both acute and chronic pain.

Classification of Pain

Pain has been classified into three major types:

1. **Pricking pain.** Pain caused by a needle, pin prick, skin cut, etc. - evokes an acute pricking quality burning pain sensation carried fast by the A delta fibers. The pain is exactly localized and of short duration. Pricking pain is also called fast pain. Pricking pain is present in all individuals and is a useful and necessary component of our sensory receptor.
2. **Burning pain or soreness pain.** Pain caused by inflammation, burned skin, etc., is carried by the C fibers (slowly conducted pain nerve fibers). This type of pain is a more diffuse, slower to onset, and longer in duration. It is an irritating and intolerable pain, which is not distinctly localized.
3. **Aching pain** is a tender pain. This pain arises mainly from the viscera and somatic deep structures. Aching pain is not clearly localized and is an annoying and intolerable pain. Aching pain is carried by the C fibers from the deep structures to the spinal cord.

Sources of Pain

Somatic Pain

Somatic pain can be classified as either: 1) cutaneous, superficial or peripheral pain and 2) deep pain.

1. **Cutaneous, Superficial or Peripheral Pain.** Pain that arises from the skin and muscles or peripheral nerves themselves. In general, this pain has two components, the initial response (a) followed by later response (b). These signals are transmitted via different pathway.
    A. Pricking pain reaches the CNS via neospinothalamic tract (i.e., LST) to the VPL (or VPM) and to the SCI.
    B. Burning and soreness pain resulting from tissue damage reaches the CNS via the paleospinothalamic tract (AST) and archispinothalamic tract to brain stem nuclei and to PF-CM complex, etc.
2. **Deep pain.** This pain originates from joint receptors tendons and deep fascia (i.e., deep structures). The quality of deep pain is dull, aching or burning. Deep pain is accompanied by a clear autonomic response associated with sweating and nausea, changes in blood pressure and heart rate.

Visceral Pain

In the visceral organs, nociceptors respond to mechanical stimulation such as pressure, tissue damage, and chemical stimulation. Most noxious information carried by visceral afferents does not give rise to conscious sensation. Visceral pain is diffuse, less precisely graded and typically accompanied by slowing of the heart, lowered blood pressure, cold sweats and nausea. It conveys also hunger, thirst, electrolyte imbalance, irregulation in the respiratory and circulatory systems.

Thalamic Pain

Stroke or occlusion in the thalamogeniculate artery (a branch of the posterior cerebral artery), which supplies the latero-posterior half of the thalamus, can result in a thalamic lesion, which is often accompanied by neurologic conditions several months after the initial event. The condition is associated with a crushing intracranial pain in the contralateral side of the thalamic lesion and sensory loss. In some cases, severe facial pain is experienced without any sensory loss. The pain resulting from an intracranial lesion is also termed "central pain."

Lesions in the spinothalamic tract can induce alteration of sensory, motor and endocrine components because of the functional diversity of the thalamus. Patient with this syndrome experience spontaneous aching and burning pain in body regions where sensory stimuli normally do not lead to pain. Because the brain and the spinal cord do not contain nociceptors, the pathological process presumably directly stimulates nociceptive pathways, or it prevents the activation of the pain suppression pathways. This condition is known also as **thalamic pain** syndrome or Dejerive-Roussy syndrome.

Neuropathic Pain

Neuropathic pain is a sharp, shooting and crushing pain. It is a persistent pain that originates from functional changes occurring in the CNS secondary to peripheral nerve injury. Once the nerve is damaged, the damaged nerve evokes sustained activation of nociceptors and/or nociceptive afferents. The neuropathic pain is due to an abnormal activation of the nociceptive system without specifically stimulating the nociceptors. The sensitization of the nervous system following injury is a factor in neuropathic pain.

Referred Pain

Referred pain is a painful sensation that present to the other site compared to the injured one. The pain is not localized to the site of its cause but instead is localized to a distant site. One possible exception is that the axons carry pain information from the injured site enter into the spinal cord by the same route as the cutaneous pain sensation axons. Within the spinal cord there is a overlap of the information on the same nocineurons. This overlap gives rise to the phenomenon of referred pain.

Pain classification based on onset:

Acute pain arises from activation of nociceptors for a limited time and is not associated with significant tissue damage (e.g., a pin prick).

Chronic Pain

Chronic pain is prolonged pain lasting for months or longer that arises from tissue injury, inflammation, nerve damage, tumor growth, lesion or occlusion of blood vessels. Chronic or inflammatory pain can sensitize the nervous system, evoking chemical, functional, and even structural changes that serve to "prime the pain-processing pump". In some cases, the pain persists long after the injury heals, but there is no treatment that will excrete the pain.

Sensitization

A classical phenomenon to describe chronic pain is called **sensitization**. Prolong noxious stimulation, nearby silent nociceptive neurons that previously were unresponsive to stimulation, now become responsive. In addition, some of the chemicals produced and released at the injured site also alter the physiological properties of nociceptors. The nociceptors commence to initiate pain signals spontaneously, which cause chronic pain. In addition, weak stimuli, such as a light touch that previously had no effect on these nociceptors, will further activate the nociceptors which result in severe pain signals. This phenomenon is referred to as "peripheral sensitization." The outcome of peripheral sensitization results in a greater and more persistent bombardment of nerve impulses firing in the CNS. The persistent bombardment of nerve impulses results in long-term changes in nerve cell activity at the level of the spinal cord and higher centers in the brain. This phenomenon is referred to as "central sensitization". It looks that peripheral and central sensitization remains after the injury obviously has healed. The sensitization of nociceptive neurons after injury results from the release of different chemicals from the damaged area. It is known that substance P and calcitonin gene-related peptides are released from peripheral nerve ending which stimulate most cells to release algesic substances which further increases the pain from the injury. In contrast, central sensitization resulting from severe and persistent injury which cause prolonged release of glutamate on nociceptive dorsal horn cells, this constant glutamate release via G protein dependant phosphorylation cascades results in opening of postsynaptic ion channels gated by the NMDA receptors. This phenomenon is also termed "wind up." This activation produces hyperexcitability of the dorsal horn cells and causes "central sensitization." Pain experts now agree that treating chronic pain early and aggressively yields the best results and prevents patients from developing physical and psychological conditions that could worsen the pain.

Pain Receptors

Pain is termed nociceptive (nocer– to injure or to hurt), and nociceptive means sensitive to noxious stimuli. Noxious stimuli are stimuli that elicit tissue damage and activate nociceptors.

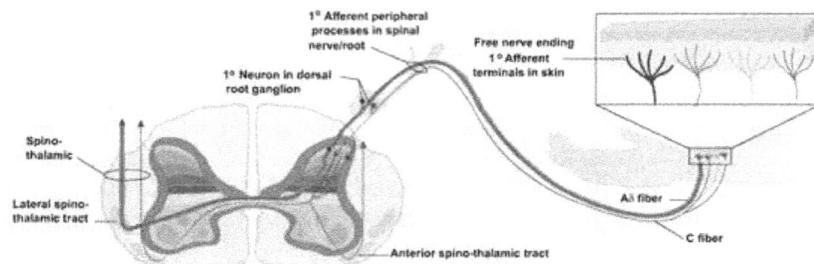

Figure 1: Different nociceptors/free nerve endings and the fibers carrying pain sensation from the nociceptors to the spinal cord.

Nociceptors are receptors that detect signals from injured tissue and also indirectly respond to chemicals released from the injured tissue. Nociceptors are free nerve endings present in the skin, muscle, joints, bone and viscera. The nerve endings contain channels that sense and detect damage called as transient receptor potential (TRP). They convert noxious stimuli into receptor potentials, which initiate action potential in the nerve fibers. This action potential is then carried to the spinal cord making a synaptic connection in lamina I and/or II. The cell of nociceptors is mainly present in the dorsal root and trigeminal ganglia. Nociceptors are not found inside the central nervous system.

Nociceptors doesn't possess a uniform sensitivity. They fall in several categories, depending on nociceptors responses to mechanical, thermal, and/or chemical stimulation presented in the damage, tumor, and/or inflammation.

- **Skin Nociceptors.** Skin nociceptors can be divided into four functional categories. The first is termed as high threshold mechano-nociceptors. These respond to intense mechanical stimulation such as pinching, cutting or stretching. The second type is the thermal nociceptors, which respond to the mechanical stimuli as well as to thermal stimuli. The third type is categorized as chemical nociceptors, which respond only to chemical substances. A fourth type is the polymodal nociceptors, which respond to high intensity stimuli, as mechanical, thermal and to chemical substances like the previous three types.
- **Joint Nociceptors.** The joint capsules and ligaments found to contain high-threshold mechanoreceptors, polymodal nociceptors. Many fibers innervating these endings in the capsule contain neuropeptides, such as substance P and calcitonin gene-related peptide (CGRP). Discharge of such peptides is conceived to play a role in the development of inflammatory arthritis.
- **Silent Nociceptors.** The "silent" nociceptors are present in the skin and deep tissues. These are normally unresponsive to any noxious mechanical stimulation, but become responsive to mechanical stimulation during inflammation. Possible explanation of the "awakening" phenomenon can be the continuous stimulation from the damaged tissue which reduces the threshold of the nociceptors and causes them to respond. The activation of the set nociceptors may cause the induction of hyperalgesia, central sensitization, and allodynia. Many visceral nociceptors are silent nociceptors.
- **Visceral Nociceptors.** Visceral organs contain mechanical pressure, temperature, chemical and silent nociceptors. The nociceptors are scattered, with variation of several millimeters between them, and in some organs, there can be several centimeters between each nociceptors. Many of the visceral nociceptors are silent. The noxious information from visceral organs and skin are carried to the CNS in different pathways.

Activation of any of the nociceptors, initiates the process pain experience. These receptors relay information to the central nervous system regarding the intensity and location of the noxious stimulus.

Factors that Activate Nociceptors

Nociceptors respond when a stimulus causes tissue damage, such as that resulting from strong mechanical pressure, extreme heat, etc. The damaged tissue results in a release of substances as well as from new substances synthesized at the site of the injury. Some of these substances activate the TRP channels which in turn initiate action potentials. These substances include:

1. **Globulin and protein kinases.** It has been suggested that damaged tissue releases globulin and protein kinases, which are believed to be amongst the most active pain-producing substances.
2. **Arachidonic acid.** Arachidonic acid is one of the chemicals released during tissue damage. It is then metabolized into prostaglandin (and cytokines). The action of the prostaglandins is mediated through a G protein, protein kinase A cascade. The prostaglandins block the potassium efflux released from nociceptors following damage, which results in additional depolarization. This makes the nociceptors more sensitive.
3. **Histamine.** Tissue damage stimulates the mast cells to release histamine to the surrounding area. Histamine excites the nociceptors. Minute subcutaneous injections of histamine elicit pain.
4. **Nerve growth factor (NGF).** Inflammation or tissue damage triggers the release of NGF. NGF then binds to TrkA receptors on the surfaces of nociceptors leading to their activation. Minute subcutaneous injections of NGF elicit pain.
5. **Substance P (SP) and Calcitonin gene-related peptide (CGRP)** are released by injury. Inflammation of damaged tissue also results in SP and CGRP release, which excites nociceptors. Both peptides produce vasodilatation, which results in the spread of edema around the initial damage.
6. **Potassium - K$^+$.** Most tissue damage results in an increase in extracellular K$^+$. There is a good correlation between pain intensity and local K$^+$ concentration.
7. **Serotonin (5-HT), acetylcholine (ACh), low pH (acidic) solution, and ATP.** These substances are released with tissue damage. Subcutaneous injections of minute qualities of these products excite nociceptors.

Pain Pathways

The ascending pathways that mediate pain consist of three different tracts: the neospinothalamic tract, the paleospinothalamic tract and the archispinothalamic tract. The first-order neurons are located in the dorsal root ganglion (DRG) for all three pathways. Each pain tract originates in different spinal cord regions and ascends to terminate in different areas in the CNS.

- **Neospinothalamic Tract**

  The **neospinothalamic tract** has few synapses and establishes the classical lateral spinothalamic tract (LST). The first-order nociceptive neurons (in the DRG) make synaptic connections in Rexed layer I neurons (marginal zone). Axons from layer I neurons intersecting in the anterior white commissure, at approximately the same level they enter the cord, and ascend in the contralateral anterolateral quadrant. Most of the pain fibers from the lower extremity and the body below the neck terminate in the ventroposterolateral (VPL) nucleus and ventroposteroinferior (VPI) nucleus of the thalamus, which serves as a relay station that sends the signals to the primary cortex. The VPL is thought to mainly be concerned with discriminatory functions. The VPL sends axons to the primary somatosensory cortex (SCI).
  The first-order nociceptive neurons from the head, face and intraoral structures have somata in the trigeminal ganglion. Trigeminal fibers enter the pons, descend to the medulla and make synaptic connections in the spinal trigeminal nucleus, cross the midline and ascend as trigeminothalamic tract . The A delta fibers terminate in the ventroposteromedial (VPM) thalamus, and the C fibers terminate in the parafasciculus (PF) and centromedian (CM) thalamus (PF-CM complex). The PF-CM complex is located within the intralaminar thalamus and are known also as intralaminar (IL) nuclei. All of the neospinothalamic fibers terminating in VPL and VPM are somatotopically oriented and from there send axons that synapse on the primary somatosensory cortex (SC I - Brodman areas 1 & 2). This pathway is responsible for

the immediate awareness of a painful sensation and for awareness of the exact location of the painful stimulus.

- **Paleospinothalamic Pathway**

  The **paleospinothalamic tract** is phylogenetically old. The majority of the first-order nociceptive neurons make synaptic connections in Rexed layer II (substantia gelatinosa) and the second-order neurons make synaptic connections in laminae IV-VIII. The second-order neurons also receive input from mechanoreceptors and thermoreceptors. The nerve cells that furnish the paleospinothalamic tract are multireceptive or wide dynamic range nociceptors. Most of their axons cross and ascend in the spinal cord primarily in the anterior region and thus called the anterior spinal thalamic tract (AST). These fibers contain several tracts. Each of them makes a synaptic connection in different locations: 1) in the mesencephalic reticular formation (MFR) and in the periaqueductal gray (PAG), and they are also called spinoreticular tract; 2) in the tectum, and these fibers are known as the spinotectal or spinomedullary tract; 3) in the PF-CM complex (IL) and they are known as the spinothalamic tract. The above three fiber tracts are known also as the paleospinothalamic tract. The innervations of these three tracts is bilateral because some of the ascending fibers do not cross to the opposite side of the cord. From the PF and CM complex, these fibers synapse bilaterally in the somatosensory cortex (SC II-Brodman area 3). The paleospinothalamic pathway also activates brain stem nuclei which are the origin of descending pain suppression pathway regulating noxious input at the spinal cord level.

  The multisynaptic tracts which course via the reticular formation also project to the PF-CM (IL) complex. There are extensive connections between the IL and the limbic areas such as the cingulate gyrus and the insular cortex, which is thought to be involved in processing the emotional components of pain. That is to say, the insular cortex integrates the sensory input with the cortical cognitive components to elicit the response to the sensation. The limbic structures, in turn, project to the hypothalamus and initiate visceral responses to pain. The intralaminar nuclei also projects to the frontal cortex, which in turn projects to the limbic structures where the emotional response to pain is mediated.

- **Archispinothalamic Pathway**

  The **archispinothalamic tract** is a multisynaptic diffuse tract or pathway and is phylogenetically the oldest tract that carries noxious information. The first-order nociceptive neurons make synaptic connections in Rexed layer II (substantia gelatinosa) and ascend to laminae IV to VII. From lamina IV to VII, fibers ascend and descend in the spinal cord via the multisynaptic propriospinal pathway surrounding the grey matter to synapse with cells in the MRF-PAG area. Further multisynaptic diffuse pathways ascend to the intralaminar (IL) areas of the thalamus (i.e., PF-CM complex) and also send collaterals to the hypothalamus and to the limbic system nuclei. These fibers mediate visceral, emotional and autonomic reactions to pain.

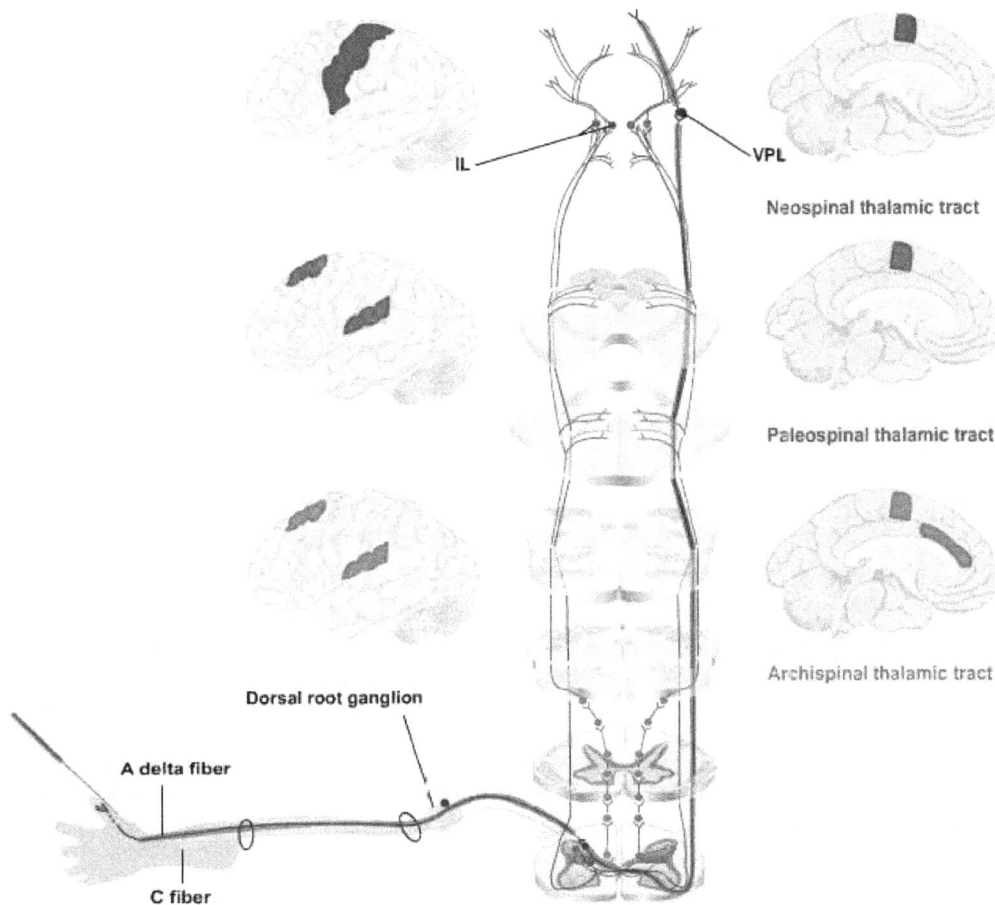

Figure 2: Summary of the three pathways carrying pain sensation.

Pain Modulation

Most, if not all, ailments of the body cause pain. Pain is interpreted and perceived in the brain. Pain is modulated by two primary types of drugs that work on the brain: analgesics and anesthetics. The term analgesic refers to a drug that relieves pain without loss of consciousness. The term central anesthesia refers to a drug that depresses the CNS. It is characterized by the absence of all perception of sensory modalities, including loss of consciousness without loss of vital functions.

- **Endogenous Opioids**

  Opioidergic neurotransmission is found throughout the brain and spinal cord and appears to influence many CNS functions, including nociception, card ovascular functions, thermoregulation, respiration, neuroendocrine functions, neuroimmune functions, food intake, sexual activity, aggressive locomotor behavior as well as learning and memory. Opioids exert marked effects on mood and motivation and produce euphoria.

  Three classes of **opioid receptors** have been identified: μ-mu, δ-delta and κ-kappa. All three classes are widely distributed in the brain. The opioid peptides modulate nociceptive input in two ways:

  - block neurotransmitter release by inhibiting Ca^{2+} influx into the presynaptic terminal,
  - open potassium channels, which hyperpolarizes neurons and inhibits spike activity.

  They act on various receptors in the brain and spinal cord. The several types of opioid receptors are distributed differently within the central and peripheral nervous system. Central or peripheral terminals of nociceptive afferent fibers contain opiate receptors where exogenous and endogenous opioids could act to modulate the ability to transmit nociceptive information. Moreover, high densities of opiate receptors are found in periaqueductal gray (PAG), nucleus raphe magnus (NRM), and dorsal raphe (DR) in the rostral ventral medulla, in the spinal cord, caudate nucleus (CN), septal nucleus, hypothalamus, habenula and hippocampus.

Gate Control theory

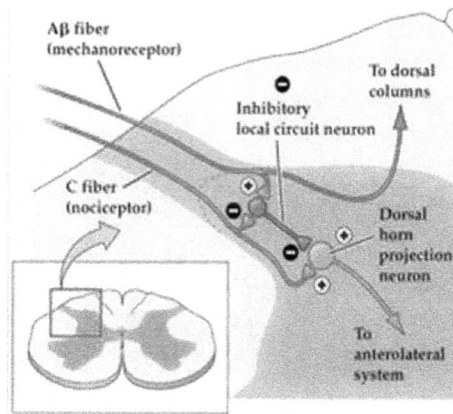

Figure 3: Pain Gait Mechanism

The first pain modulatory mechanism called the **"Gate Control" theory** was proposed by Melzack and Wall in the mid 1960s. The theory suggests that collaterals of the large sensory fibers carrying cutaneous sensory input activate inhibitory interneurons, which inhibit (modulate) pain transmission information carried by the pain fibers. Non-noxious input suppresses pain, or sensory input "closes the gate" to noxious input. The gate theory predicts that at the spinal cord level, non-noxious stimulation will produce presynaptic inhibition on dorsal root nociceptor fibers that synapse on nociceptors spinal neurons (T), and this presynaptic inhibition will block incoming noxious information from reaching the CNS (i.e., will close the gate to incoming noxious information).

Descending Pain Suppression Mechanism

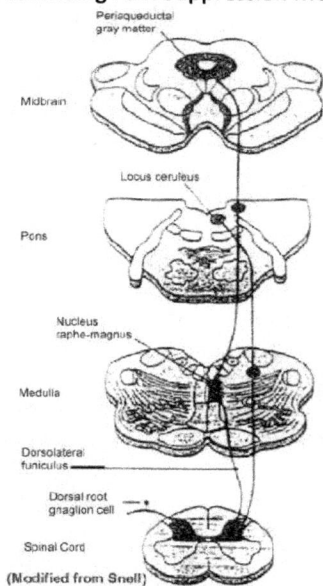

Figure 4: Descending pain modulatory circuit

The primary ascending pain fibers (the A δ and C fibers) reach the dorsal horn of the spinal cord from peripheral sites to innervate the nociceptor neurons in Rexed laminae I & II. Cells from Rexed lamina II make synaptic connections in Rexed layers IV to VII. Cells, especially in laminae I and VII of the dorsal horn, give rise to ascending spinothalamic tracts. At the spinal level, opiate receptors are located at the presynaptic ends of the nocineurons and at the interneural level layers IV to VII in the dorsal horn. Activation of opiate receptors at the interneuronal level produces hyperpolarization of the neurons, which result in the inhibition of firing and the release of substance P, a neurotransmitter involved in pain transmission, thereby blocking pain transmission. The circuit that consists of the periaqueductal gray (PAG) matter in the upper brain stem, the locus coeruleus (LC), the nucleus raphe magnus (NRM) and the nucleus reticularis gigantocellularis (Rgc) contributes to the descending pain suppression pathway, which inhibits incoming pain information at the spinal cord level.

The opioids interact with the opiate receptors at different CNS levels. These opiate receptors are the normal target sites for neurotransmitters and endogenous opiates such as the endorphins and enkephalins. As a result of binding at the receptor in subcortical sites, secondary changes which lead to a change in the electrophysiological properties of these neurons and modulation of the ascending pain information.

It was found that noxious stimulation excites neurons in the nucleus reticularis gigantocellularis (RGC). The nucleus RGC innervates both the PAG and NRM. The PAG sends axons to NRM, and neurons in NRM send their axons to the spinal cord.

Opiate receptors have also been found in the dorsal horn of the spinal cord, mainly in Rexed laminae I, II, and V, and these spinal opiate receptors mediate inhibitory effects on dorsal horn neurons transmitting nociceptive information. In addition, there are ascending connections from the PAG and raphe nuclei to PF-CM complex. These thalamic areas are part of the ascending pain modulation at the diencephalon level.

Myofascial Trigger Points

Myofascial pain syndrome (MPS) is a common source of frustration among health care practitioner. It involves as much as 85 percent of general population. As the name suggest it is the collection of sensory, motor, and autonomic symptoms which includes local/referred pain, decreased ROM and weakness. While myofascial pain syndrome is complex in its presentation, the onset and persistence of myofascial pain syndrome are known to be caused by myofascial trigger points. In patients, myofascial trigger points present as focal areas in muscle that appear stiff and hyper contracted and are painful particularly when palpated. Despite the causal association of myofascial trigger points with the underlying physiology of myofascial pain syndrome, the mechanisms that induce the onset and maintenance of myofascial trigger points are unknown.

Myofascial pain syndrome is caused by myofascial trigger points which are identified by palpation as discrete foci of hyper contracted areas within a muscle. Clinically, myofascial trigger points are defined as active or latent. An active myofascial trigger point is recognized as eliciting spontaneous pain as well as pain, referred pain, and motor or autonomic symptoms on palpation. These include an impaired range of motion, muscle weakness, and loss of coordination. In contrast, latent myofascial trigger points upon palpation/compression cause pain, a local twitch response, and referred pain. In fact they may display all the symptoms of an active trigger point to a lesser degree. For example latent trigger points may have associated autonomic symptoms with pain and their presence results in a limited range of motion, muscle fatigability, and muscle weakness as in the active presentation. This makes latent trigger points a significant concern also.

It is important to distinguish between myofascial pain and neuropathic pain. While myofascial pain originates at the muscle, neuropathic pain results from an injury to or malfunction of the peripheral or central nervous system. There are myriad different pain syndromes and chronic pain disorder that fall into the category of neuropathic pain. Myofascial pain, on the other hand, is thought to originate at the trigger point in the taut band of muscle. In order to begin to gain mechanistic insights into the mechanisms of myofascial trigger points, it is helpful to consider aspects of skeletal muscle physiology.

Excitation-Contraction Coupling: the neural activation of the muscle cell initiate contraction and subsequent relaxation of the muscle fiber. Skeletal muscle, like cardiac muscle, is called striated muscle because it has a banded appearance within the single myocyte due to repeated pattern of contractile units termed as sarcomeres. Contraction of skeletal muscle is controlled by motor neurons and graded by motor units, which are the collection of muscle fibers innervated by a single motor neuron. At the neuromuscular junction (i.e., the interface between a motor neuron and a single muscle fiber), a motor neuron action potential starts the release of acetylcholine from the presynaptic nerve terminals. Acetylcholine then diffuses across the synaptic cleft to activate nicotinic acetylcholine receptors in the postsynaptic membrane. Muscle contraction occurs when the summation of acetylcholine receptor activation reaches the threshold to trigger voltage dependent sodium channel activation in the sarcolemma outside the neuromuscular junction and subsequent action potential generation and depolarization of the muscle fiber. The clearance of acetylcholine from the synaptic cleft by acetyl-cholinesterase resets the process for subsequent activation.

The contraction of the muscle fiber is triggered by action potential transmission deep within the muscle fiber through sarcolemmal membrane infoldings termed as transverse tubules (t-tubules). Anatomic specialization within the t-tubule is seen at the triad where the t-tubule is flanked by the calcium storage organelle, the sarcoplasmic reticulum. The membrane depolarization accompanying the arrival of the action potential at the triadic space within the t-tubule, activates voltage dependent L-type calcium channels in the transverse tubular membrane. Type I ryanodine receptors are located in the sarcoplasmic reticulum in close proximity to the L-type channels and physical coupling between the type I ryanodine receptors and the L-type calcium channels (they either directly or through accessory proteins cause the ryanodine receptors to undergo a conformational change and open releasing calcium into the myoplasm).

This transient rise in calcium binds to troponin on the actin thin filament, which relieves the inhibition on actin for binding by the contractile protein myosin. The calcium dependent interaction of actin and myosin occurs through the formation of strongly bound myosin crossbridges to actin. Force is then generated through ATP (adenosine triphosphate) dependent processes. Critical to this process is ATP hydrolysis that provides energy for the enzymatic activity of the myosin head which generates a single articulation of the myosin head and molecular movement of actin past myosin which shortens the sarcomere. The rebinding of a new ATP is then needed to relieve the strongly bound actin and myosin. In this process, muscle shortening occurs at a rate dependent on the speed of myosin's enzymatic activity and the resultant force and power output is the ensemble of the crossbridge cycle (i.e., attachment-myofilament sliding-detachment) of all myosin heads in each muscle. The crossbridge cycle is therefore calcium and ATP dependent and maintained as long as calcium and ATP remain high in the cytoplasm. In fact, a depletion of ATP while calcium is elevated results in the inability of crossbridge detachment and the formation of the "rigor bond" which leads to the stiffness seen postmortem.

Subsequent to the calcium release into the myoplasm, the sarcoendoplasmic reticulum ATPase (SERCA) works to isolate calcium back into the sarcoplasmic reticulum, again via ATP dependent enzymatic activity. Subsequent to a brief activation (~5msec) by a single action potential, troponin, SERCA, and a host of other calcium binding proteins compete for calcium such that a brief force transient is realised (i.e., twitch). Grading force production at the single muscle fibre is then produced by delivering action potentials at higher frequencies (i.e., repetitive firing of the motor unit) resulting in pulses of calcium release that progressively increase myoplasmic calcium concentration.

Energetics: The molecule ATP is the vital energy source for muscle function. The metabolic processes that generate ATP use carbohydrates, fatty acids and sometimes amino acids as their primary substrate. Carbohydrates are converted to glucose which enters the glycolysis pathway in the cell cytoplasm. The end product of this process is pyruvate which is converted to acetyl CoA by pyruvate dehydrogenase in the mitochondria. The β-oxidation of fatty acids results in formation of acetyl CoA. Acetyl CoA enters the tricarboxylic acid cycle (Krebs cycle) that takes place in the mitochondria. Amino acids are converted to other Krebs cycle intermediates and enter the cycle at different point. The Krebs cycle produces the reducing equivalents NADH and $FADH_2$ that enter the electron transport chain. The electron transport chain uses the energy contained in the reducing equivalents to pump protons out of the mitochondria producing an electrochemical gradient (pH gradient and membrane potential) that is used to make ATP. The electron transport chain consumes oxygen during proton pumping resulting in the term oxidative phosphorylation to describe the entire process that transfers the energy in the reducing equivalents to ATP. Hence, the mitochondria in the myocytes provide the ATP needed for contraction. Skeletal muscles contain approximately 1–12% mitochondria by volume depending upon the particular muscle. Muscles with higher energy demand have higher mitochondrial content.

Reactive Oxygen Species: Striated muscle generates reactive oxygen species (ROS) which acts which modulates a host of biochemical processes including glucose uptake, gene expression, calcium indicating, and contractility through the targeted modification of specific protein residues. In striated muscle, contractile activity increases ROS indicating which leads to physiologic adaptation; however, in pathological conditions, ROS indicating is often in excess where it contributes to contractile dysfunction and myopathy.

Striated muscle generates superoxide as the primary ROS. Superoxide is generated by the addition of a single electron to ground state oxygen. Superoxide is a highly reactive, unstable species that is rapidly converted by superoxide dismutase (SOD) to hydrogen peroxide (H_2O_2), a weaker but more stable oxidant. H_2O_2 is highly diffusible within and between cells, activates multiple signaling pathways, and is decomposed by either catalase or glutathione peroxidase to water and oxygen.

The most well described source for superoxide production is the mitochondria where superoxide is produced within the electron transport chain (ETC). Recent work estimates that, at rest, the percentage of the ROS generated by electron flow through the ETC is low (<1%). During sustained vigorous contractile activity, however, where mitochondrial function increases >50-fold, the magnitude of superoxide release is modestly increased, only a small amount (~2–4-fold) over resting levels.

Two additional ROS sources are operant in muscle and yet are likely to be of significance only in disease or high stress conditions. The enzyme xanthine oxidase (XO) has been shown to produce superoxide in response to contractile activity in rodent muscle. Available evidence however supports either a vascular source of XO generated superoxide due to contractile shear stress or an increase in

XO activity secondary to anaerobic metabolism that increases the availability of XO substrates. Superoxide is also produced by phospholipase A2 (PLA2) dependent processes with a Ca^{2+}-independent PLA2 contributing to ROS production under resting conditions, whereas a Ca^{2+}-dependent PLA2 may contribute to ROS production during contraction when cytosolic $[Ca^{2+}]$ is elevated. While XO or PLA2 sources of ROS are unlikely to play a role in the sustained ROS production at rest or during dynamic contractions, each supports a mechanism to increase superoxide following exhaustive/fatiguing contractions or sustained contractures where anaerobic metabolism predominates.

Recent work in striated muscle by Ward and coworkers and others has implicated Nicotinamide Adenine Dinucleotide Phosphate Oxidase 2 (NADPH oxidase; NOX) as the major source of superoxide ROS during repetitive contraction. NOX is a multimeric enzymatic complex that generates superoxide by transferring electrons from NADPH to oxygen. Several NOX isoforms are expressed in striated muscle and located within the sarcoplasmic reticulum, the sarcolemma, and the transverse tubules. Striated muscle cells express NOX2 and 4 which each bind $p22^{phox}$, a small subunit essential for enzyme activity. NOX4 is component, active and does not require association with regulatory subunits, with regulation thought to occur mainly by changes in expression level. Therefore NOX4 likely contributes to the basal rate of ROS production in the myocyte. In contrast, NOX2 (also known as gp9) is activated by specific agonists (e.g. G-protein coupled receptor agonists such as angiotensin II, growth factors, and cytokines) and mechanical/contractile stress, which induce the association of regulatory subunits ($p47^{phox}$, $p67^{phox}$ $p40^{phox}$, and Rac1) and activation of the enzyme.

The mechanosensitivity of NOX2 has recently gathered much attention. The production of reactive oxygen species by NADPH oxidase is regulated by the small Rho like GTPase protein Rac1. The Rac1 protein activity is regulated by microtubules and the actin cytoskeleton. During mechanical stress such as the stretching/twisting of airway smooth muscle cells, the cytoskeleton deforms and activates Rac1. This response is disrupted if myosin II tension is blocked with blebbistatin, f-actin is disrupted with cytochalasin D, or the microtubules are disrupted with colchicine. This mechanism is also present in skeletal muscle where mechanical stretching induces ROS production by NOX2. This mechanoactivation of NOX2 dependent ROS production has been recently shown to be critical to the pathogenic calcium and ROS indicating in Duchenne muscular dystrophy.

Myofascial Trigger Points

Myofascial "trigger points", coined in the 1950's by Dr. Janet Travell and Dr. David Simon, are commonly defined in clinical practice as the presence of deep local tenderness at a nodule in a palpable taut band of muscle which, when stimulated, can cause a referred pattern of pain. Trigger points can produce referred pain to other musculature spontaneously or with manual compression to the site within the muscle. Myofascial trigger points can present in individuals through occupational or athletic activities, where postural deficiencies, muscle imbalances, and overuse injuries can occur.

Anatomy of Myofascial Trigger Points

Voluntary muscle contraction is controlled by the central nervous system. Motor centers in the brain sends signals, in the form of action potentials, to anterior horn alpha motor neurons that innervate extrafusal muscle fibers. Contraction of muscle fibers occurs when the neurotransmitter acetylcholine is released into the neuromuscular junction from presynaptic clefts and binds to receptors on the muscle cell membrane at the motor end plate zone. The binding of acetylcholine causes calcium to enter the muscle cell. As a result of calcium troponin proteins move the myosin heads up the actin molecule. This flow of events

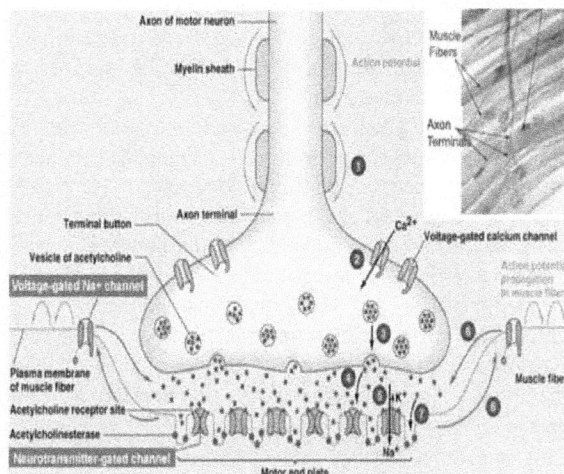

Figure 5: Axon of motor neuron at neuromuscular junction

causes the sarcomere, the functional unit of the muscle, to shorten and contract.

Trigger points (TrPs) are located at the center, of belly, of the muscle in the motor endplate zone. Motor nerves in this zone enter a muscle and divide into branches each with a terminal claw-like motor endplate embedded in the surface of a muscle fiber. Muscle fibers with active TrPs contract to form a distinctive taut band. Normal muscle fibers have sarcomeres of equal length. Muscle fibers containing contraction knots, or "fusiform swellings", have shortened sarcomeres at the site and lengthened muscle fibers on either side. Neurovascular bundles associated with TrP sites contain a motor axon with branching motor nerve endings that have terminal motor endplates with contractile "knots". Nociceptive and proprioceptive sensory afferents, blood vessels, and associated sympathetic fibers are also found within the bundle.

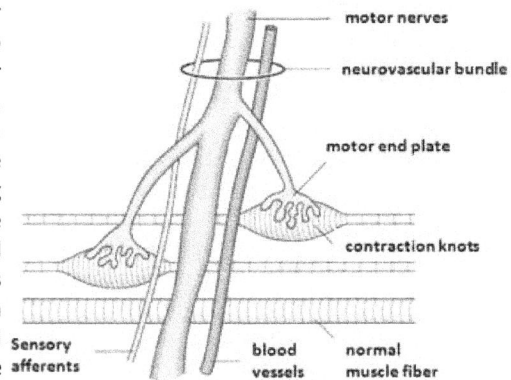

Figure 6: Structures involved in MTrP

Trigger Point Pathophysiology

Trigger points can be found in skin and periosteum but are most prevalent in muscle tissue. There are several theories surrounding the underlying causes of TrP's. One of the widely excepted mechanisms is the Motor Endplate Hypothesis which identifies dysfunction in the region of extrafusal motor endplates as a primary cause of myofascial TrPs. It is suspected that when pain develops at the site of a TrP, sensitized nociceptor sensory afferents release calcitonin gene-related peptides which then cause an increased rate of release of acetylcholine from motor endplates further contracting muscle fibers. Though disbelief still surrounds this mechanism of TrP formation, electromyography (EMG) studies have demonstrated that spontaneous electrical activity found at TrP sites correspond to abnormal patterns of motor end plate electrical activity brought about by excessive release of acetylcholine.

Active MTPs are also the main peripheral pain generator in generalized musculoskeletal pain disorders, such as fibromyalgia and whiplash syndrome. MTPs are the targets for dry needling and other pain therapies. Indeed, MTP anesthetization decreases both pain intensity and central sensitization in local pain and generalized pain conditions.

Registered with intramuscular needle electromyography (EMG) when the muscle is at rest, spontaneous electrical activity (SEA) is one of the characteristics of MTP. SEA is dysfunctional extrafusal motor endplate potential (EPP), rather than from the gamma motor units within muscle spindle.

Prolonged or unaccustomed exercise, acute and chronic mechanical and electrical trauma and prolonged ischemia lead to cell membrane damage which is the initial event in muscle damage. Following cell membrane damage, influx of $Ca2+$ is increased, leading to $Ca2+$ overload. As a result, calpains and phospholipase A2 may be activated; production of reactive oxygen species may be increased; and mitochondrial $Ca2+$ may be overloaded, thereby further worsening the damage in a self-reinforcing manner. In addition to $Ca2+$ overload, an increase in $Na+$ permeability and the accompanying increase in $Na+$ influx also induce membrane depolarization. Thus, mechanical trauma causes direct injury to the cellular membrane, causing $Ca2+$ and $Na+$ to flood the injured tissue. The $Ca2+$ overload contributes to the initiation of spontaneous activity at motor endplate. The localized $Na+$ conductance change in the membrane of the active muscle fiber may also lead to the initiation of spontaneous action potentials at motor endplate. The acetylcholine (Ach) released at a motor unit associated with MTP may be also modulated by other ion channels.

EPP, which is a local depolarization of the muscle fibers, spreads a short distance along the muscle fibers, with a decrement of about 50-75 per cent per millimeter. If the EPP exceeds a certain critical level (by summation of successive EPPs), endplate spikes are initiated, explaining the clinical phenomenon that SEA associated with MTP, is registered only in a localized spot in the muscle with intramuscular needle EMG. Enormously increased abnormal spontaneous release of Ach produces the SEA. SEA is a combination of endplate noise and endplate spikes with action potentials generated by sufficient amounts of spontaneously released Ach. Studies in MTP animal models also show that the SEA is significantly decreased by botulinum toxin which inhibits the release of acetylcholine at the neuromuscular junction.

Both extrafusal (alpha motor unit) and intrafusal fibers (gamma motor unit within muscle spindle) are cholinergically innervated; the decrease in the SEA following botulinum toxin application cannot differentiate the source of SEA from the alpha motor unit or from the gamma motor unit. The discharge patterns of static and dynamic gamma motoneurones contribute to the control of locomotion, but contraction of the intrafusal muscle fibers does not contribute to the force of muscle contraction. Muscle force is positively correlated with the amplitude of EMG during dynamic contraction. Analysis of the motor behaviors of an MTP clearly shows that intramuscular EMG activity at an MTP (SEA) exhibits similar motor behavior to the surface EMG activity over an MTP and is also similar to the intramuscular and surface EMG over a non-MTP during voluntary muscle contractions in the upper trapezius muscle, suggesting that the SEA activity during movement contributes to the muscle force production. Thus, this motor behavior of MTP indicates that the SEA originates from the extrafusal motor endplate but not from the intrafusal motor endplate. No electrophysiological methods are currently available to record electrical activities from intrafusal motor endplate directly in the muscle. Instead, efferent discharges of intrafusal motor endplate are indirectly assessed with microneurography recorded from peripheral nerve fibers in animals and humans. Efferent discharges of intrafusal motor endplate are uncorrelated with any activation of extrafusal muscle fibers in humans though intrafusal motor units are generally spontaneously active. However, the SEA may be recorded with intramuscular EMG in humans and originates from extrafusal motor endplate in several pathophysiological conditions; including MTPs. SEA at MTPs may play a significant role in the induction of pain.

Initiation of Myofascial Trigger Points

A clear mechanistic description for the initiation of a myofascial trigger point does not currently exist. Trigger points are thought to occur as a result of muscle overuse or muscle trauma or psychological stress. Examples include trigger points arising secondary to muscle overload in worksite tasks or activities of daily living such as lifting heavy objects or sustained repetitive activities. In these cases, poor ergonomics, improper postural positioning, deconditioned muscle, and fatigue have been associated with the development myofascial trigger point. While muscle conditioning has been shown to reduce the incidence, the occurrence of myofascial trigger points in elite athletes suggests a threshold above which inciting events may initiate a myofascial trigger point. Psychological stress may complement these mechanisms in the development of myofascial trigger point.

Another important consideration is that, in some healthy individuals and athletes, muscle fatigue or trauma does not always result in myofascial trigger points. Instead they can result in stiffness, soreness, and pain that usually resolve themselves after a few days. This also supports a threshold for occurrence and/or possibly a cofactor that promotes the initiation of a myofascial trigger point. Here, clues to the mechanistic events that initiate myofascial trigger points may be gained from our knowledge that co morbid conditions such as aging, disease, and stress increase the incidence of myofascial trigger points. For example, myofascial trigger points are thought to underlie the spontaneous pain patter in individuals suffering from fibromyalgia. Trigger points also have been observed with an increased frequency in patients suffering from reflex sympathetic dystrophy which is thought to arise from the unique emotional and psychological condition of these patients and psychological stress in other patients. Additionally, myofascial trigger points may arise secondary to causes as certain cancer therapeutic regimens (i.e., taxanes and pacilitaxil) induce myofascial pain.

Myofascial trigger points are more common under conditions of psychological stress. In fact, myofascial trigger points display increased myogenic activity, while the adjacent muscle remained silent under psychological stress. Psychological stress results in an increase of certain hormones and increase of sympathetic neural stimulation. It is believed that the increase in hormones and sympathetic stimulation during this condition leads to increase in release of acetylcholine at the neuromuscular junction contributing to the contraction of the motor units involved in a trigger point.

Mechanisms for Persistence of Myofascial Trigger Points

The persistence of myofascial trigger points requires a self-sustaining positive feed-forward process. Simons presented the integrated hypothesis for myofascial trigger points to offer an explanation. The integrated hypothesis is a six-link chain that starts with step (1): the abnormal release of acetylcholine. This triggers step (2): increased muscle fiber tension which is seen as the taut band found in a myofascial trigger point. The taut band is thought to constrict blood flow that leads to step (3): local hypoxia. The reduced oxygen disrupts mitochondrial energy metabolism reducing ATP and leads to step (4): tissue distress and step (5): the release of sensitizing substances. These sensitizing substances lead to pain by activation of nociceptors (pain receptors) and also lead to step (6): autonomic modulation that then potentiates step (1): abnormal acetylcholine release.

More recently this hypothesis has been expanded by Gerwin and coworkers. It suggests more specific details of the feedback loop. For example, sympathetic nervous system activity augments acetylcholine release as well as the local hypoperfusion caused by the muscle contraction. The resulting ischemia/hypoxia leads to acidification (decreased pH). Experiments have shown that injections of acidic saline of pH 4 can cause muscle pain through activation of muscle pain receptors called acid-sensing ion channels (ASIC3). While this low pH is much lower than that seen during ischemia, a smaller physiological decrease in pH has been shown to activate ASIC3 channels. The prolonged ischemia/hypoxia also leads to muscle injury resulting in the release of potassium, bradykinins, cytokines, ATP, and substance P which might stimulate nociceptors in the muscle. The end result is the tenderness and pain observed with myofascial trigger points accompanied by calcitonin gene-related peptide (CGRP). Depolarization of nociceptive neurons causes the release of CGRP. CGRP inhibits acetylcholine esterase and upregulates the amount of acetylcholine receptors and release of acetylcholine. This nonquantal spontaneous acetylcholine release at the motor end plate as a result of CGRP is termed as acetylcholine leakage. This differs from the other modes of acetylcholine release such as simulation induced multiquantal release resulting in an end plate potential (EPP) and spontaneous quantal releases resulting in a miniature end plate potential (MEPP). The theory also postulates CGRP release from nerve terminals with the same targets. Furthermore, a decrease in pH can also cause an increase in acetylcholine release. The result is increased acetylcholine in the nerve terminal, synaptic cleft, and increased motor endplate potentials resulting in more contraction. The model also suggests that psychological stress also increases acetylcholine release into the neuromuscular junction.

Using microdialysis, samples of the chemical, surroundings of the muscle can be obtained. In microdialysis, a hollow needle filled with an absorbing gel and with a semipermeable membrane at its tip is inserted into the myofascial trigger point. Another is inserted into adjacent normal muscle for comparison. Ions, signaling molecules, and proteins diffuse into the gel that does not leave the needle. These are assayed upon removal of the needle. While this method allows access to the muscle interior, it cannot differentiate between the intracellular and extracellular spaces. Such experiments, hence, can give an idea of the chemical species in the muscle tissue but not specifically describe the intracellular conditions of the skeletal muscle cell.

The positive feedback loop in the above mechanism requires that there be sustained stimulation of the muscle motor unit due to increased acetylcholine release and decreased acetylcholinesterase activity. However, it appears that acetylcholine release might not be required for sustaining trigger points. In studies comparing the efficacy of motor nerve block using lidocaine injection compared to intramuscular stimulation using dry needling, the group receiving the intramuscular stimulation showed more than 40% greater improvement than did the lidocaine injection group. Furthermore, lidocaine shows a dose-dependent decrease in miniature end plate potential, acetylcholine release, and acetylcholine sensitivity. Therefore, there might be another mechanism that provides the positive feedback that sustains a myofascial trigger point. However, if the spontaneous nonquantal acetylcholine release is a direct result of CGRP, it might be too small to measure and, since it does not involve nerve depolarization, would be unaffected by lidocaine.

New Mechanistic Theory for Myofascial Trigger Points

The current theory for the mechanisms behind myofascial pain is not sufficient to fully explain the syndrome. As the myofascial trigger point appears central to the onset, and persistence of myofascial pain syndrome is still unclear, a mechanistic findings in muscle demonstrates how mechanical stress acts to trigger excess calcium release in muscle via a novel mechano-transduction pathway. With this new pathway the initiation and persistence of myofascial trigger points extends the current theories discussed above.

Initiation of a Myofascial Trigger Point

The essence of this question is what positive feedback mechanisms exist that can sustain a myofascial trigger point once initiated. The local and persistent hyper contracture of the muscle appears to be critical to the myofascial trigger point. At the cellular level, a persistent neural activation may act to initiate a local and sustained contraction; however, fatigue of the muscle would result much as in a highly trained athlete with high motivation that is eventually unable to sustain muscle activity. Rather, the local contracture of the muscle must occur secondary to the normal neuromuscular activation and arise due to regenerative feed-forward processes within the muscle cell. At the most basic level, this situation would demand a mechanism that permitted regenerative calcium release within the myofibers that escaped from the normal inhibitory processes that govern central and peripheral muscle fatigue. It would be most practical for this feed-forward mechanism to take advantage of any aberrant activity (contraction dependent mechanical stress, calcium release, and altered metabolic signaling) as an initiation trigger and as a mechanism to sustain its activity.

X-ROS signaling is a newly characterized mechanoactivated ROS-dependent indicating cascade in cardiac and skeletal muscle. In X-ROS signaling mechanical deformation of the microtubule network acts as a mechanotransduction element to activate the NADPH oxidase (NOX2) which produces ROS. The ROS oxidizes RyRs and increases their open probability resulting in increases in Ca^{2+} release from the sarcoplasmic reticulum. The Ca^{2+} mobilization resulting from mechanical stretch through this pathway is X-ROS signaling. In heart, X-ROS acts locally to affect the sarcoplasmic reticulum (SR) Ca^{2+} release channels (ryanodine receptors, ryanodine receptors) and "tunes" excitation-contraction coupling Ca^{2+} signaling during physiological behavior but can promote Ca^{2+}-dependent arrhythmias during pathology with X-ROS in excess. In skeletal muscle, X-ROS sensitizes Ca^{2+}-permeable sarcolemmal "transient receptor potential" (TRP) channels, a pathway critical for sustaining SR load during repetitive contractions. When in excess, X-ROS in skeletal muscle is maladaptive as shown in diseases such as Duchenne muscular dystrophy (DMD) and dysferlinopathy which both have altered calcium signalling as major mechanistic underpinnings. Importantly, work in DMD by Khairallah et al. suggests that the development of X-ROS (i.e., enhancement in the expression of microtubule protein and NOX2 and its resultant increase in mechanoactivated ROS) is a secondary process that is temporally associated with the severity of the disease and not a primary cause of the disease. In that regard the enhancement in X-ROS was a disease modifier that increased the severity of the disease by lowering the threshold for calcium release in the muscle.

The above mechanism proposes that excessive contraction dependent stress acts through the microtubule cytoskeletal elements to activate NADPH oxidase to produce ROS. The subsequent ROS sensitization of ryanodine receptors and sarcolemmal calcium influx channels increases myoplasmic calcium concentration and contraction leading to more stretch. Based on this model, one reason why the occurrence of myofascial trigger points may be less common in healthy individuals is due to the absence of the feed-forward trigger, excess microtubules, or NOX2 that serves to generate X-ROS. This hypothesis then proposes that the threshold for developing myofascial pain and myofascial trigger points is lower with the trigger present as a critical amount of X-ROS activity that would serve to lower the threshold for calcium release activation such that spontaneous or regenerative calcium release generation promoted can initiate the contractures which underscore the myofascial trigger point.

Myofascial trigger points are thought to occur by muscle injury and muscle overuse. In heart muscle the increased mechanical stretch and increased mechanical load underpin heart failure and result in increases in microtubule density and polymerization. Furthermore, in cardiac muscle prolonged stretching increases mitochondrial biogenesis through the focal adhesion kinase (FAK) signaling pathway. Blocking this pathway using RNAi attenuated the increase in mitochondrial biogenesis. If chronic functional overload of skeletal muscle also resulted in microtubule dependent effects, this could offer an explanation for muscle imbalances leading to functional overload of muscle such as the trapezius which is prone to myofascial trigger points and foci for myofascial pain in the upper back.

Recently, noninvasive imaging studies using doppler ultrasound or vibration elastography have been shown effective in detecting myofascial trigger points. Areas associated with myofascial trigger points are hyper echoic under ultrasound imaging having lower vibration amplitude and entropy, respectively, than that of normal muscle. This finding is consistent with increased tissue density which is indicative of a contracture or proliferation of a protein. In fact, in cardiac muscle, increasing microtubule polymerization by application of taxol increases tissue viscosity. Depolymerization of microtubules by colchicine had the opposite effect. As microtubule density has been shown to correlate with cell viscosity/stiffness, it is hypothesize that the hyperechoic regions in the ultrasound of myofascial trigger points are reflective of an increase microtubule density.

In addition to the increase of ROS production through the X-ROS mechanism, a reduced ability of the muscle cell to remove ROS most likely also plays a role in the mechanism. In normal stretching of the muscle, reactive oxygen species are removed by the normal homeostatic mechanisms. Superoxide is reduced to hydrogen peroxide by superoxide dismutase. The hydrogen peroxide is removed by catalase or glutathione oxidase and converted to water. The glutathione that is oxidized to glutathione compound is converted back to glutathione by glutathione reductase consuming NADPH in the process. The regeneration of NADPH uses the nicotinamide nucleotide transhydrogenase which requires a proton gradient and membrane potential across the mitochondrial inner membrane. The local ischemia that results from the formation of a myofascial trigger point will result in a decrease in mitochondrial membrane potential and increase in extra mitochondrial proton concentration (decreased pH). This reduces the ability of the muscle to remove reactive oxygen species and should contribute to the maintenance of high reactive oxygen species level that leads to sustained myofascial trigger points.

As mentioned previously, muscle-damaging exercise and psychological stress play a role in the initiation of myofascial trigger points. This might be due to the reduced ability of the muscle to remove ROS under these conditions. Experimental studies have shown that repeated muscle-damaging exercises results in muscle oxidative stress which includes decreased levels of glutathione and increased levels of its oxidized form, glutathione compound. Psychological stress increases mitochondrial biogenesis in the short term. On the other hand, sustained exposure to the hormones produced during psychological stress decreases mitochondrial biogenesis. Furthermore, this prolonged stress increases mitochondrial ROS production. This increased ROS production might further deplete antioxidant defense systems, increasing overall cellular reactive oxygen species levels.

What Causes a Myofascial Trigger Point to Be Painful?

Myofascial trigger points yield pain upon palpation. If they are only painful upon palpation, they are called latent. If they are painful without manipulation they are considered to be active. Given current information, there are two possible and perhaps complementary mechanisms behind the pain experienced as a result of myofascial trigger points. These two mechanisms involve the nociceptors ASIC3 (acid-sensing ion channel) and TRPV1 (transient receptor potential) channel in pain sensing neurons. These mechanisms are described below.

The local sustained contraction in a myofascial trigger point can result in restriction of local circulation which can cause the local ischemia/hypoxia and the observed changes caused by it such as increased acid accumulation resulting in a decrease in pH. In experiments in rabbit gastrocnemius muscle, the intracellular pH dropped from 7.0 to 6.6 during 4 hours of ischemia. In the extracellular fluid the pH changes from 7.3 to 6.36 during the same time period due to the accumulation of lactic acid. There are four ASIC channels: ASIC1, ASIC2, ASIC3, and ASIC4. However, only ASIC3 seems to be involved in inflammatory pain. This pH drop is enough to fully activate the nociceptive ASIC3 channels in nearby neurons. The pH changes seemed to level off due to a drop in membrane potential from -90 mV to -60 mV which resulted in increased proton extrusion.

As noted above, reactive oxygen species are produced in large amounts as a result of the mechanism of myofascial trigger points. There are several TRP (transient receptor potential) channels that respond to reactive oxygen species including TRPM2, TRPM7, TRPC5, TRPV1, and TRPA1. The TRP channels involved in pain are TRPV1–V4, TRPA1, and TRPM8. These two sets intersect at the TRPV1 channel making it a likely contributor. In fact, recent experiments have shown that reactive oxygen species can activate nociceptors in pain sensing neurons and enhance inflammatory pain. Furthermore, the TRPV1 channel is also known as the capsaicin receptor. Capsaicin applied topically has been shown to reduce myofascial pain.

Considering that the two nociceptors above most likely are involved in the sensation of pain in the environment of trigger points, the question arises—why are some trigger points latent and some active? Pain is likely felt with manipulation of trigger points as the cytoskeleton is being stretched and reactive oxygen species production increased activation of more nociceptors. Some trigger points might be active because the local extracellular reactive oxygen species concentration in the location of the TRPV1 receptors is high enough for their activation. This requires that these receptors be close enough to the trigger point. The active trigger points are likely located closer to pain receptor channels so that the receptors see high levels of protons and ROS. Hence both ASIC3 and TRPV1 channels are activated. Latent channels are farther away so that they see lower levels of ROS (which dissipates faster than the pH gradient as ROS are unstable and larger molecules). Experimental studies have indicated that pressing on a cell activates stretch-activated channels causing increases in myoplasmic calcium. This suggests that palpation might also trigger stretch-activated processes such as X-ROS signaling. Therefore, when palpated, the ROS levels might rise resulting in activation of the TRPV1 channels causing pain.

There are also other receptor channels that are located in the pain sensing neuron that are involved in the sensation of pain in myofascial pain syndrome. The bradykinin receptors (B1 and B2) are involved in inflammatory pain. Serotonin receptors likely do not depolarize the neuron due to the low levels of serotonin in tissues but instead sensitize the neurons to activation by other factors. Prostaglandin (particularly E2) also sensitizes the pain sensing neuron. The P2X3 receptors are activated by ATP and its derivatives which can be released as a result of muscle injury. Glutamate receptors might also be involved as glutamate injections have been shown to lower the pressure pain threshold in patients.

In summary, it appears that myofascial pain is likely due to a combined activation of several ligand gated ion channels in the pain sensing neuron. For example, ASIC3 and TRPV1 open as a result of increased acidity and reactive oxygen species, respectively. Any treatment for pain should address these mechanisms.

Mechanisms of local and referred muscle pain associated with MTP

Local and referred muscle pain can be consistently induced by mechanical stimulation of active MTPs. The local and referred pain from active MTPs can be recognized by the patients as their pain experience during daily activities (activity related pain) and/or at rest (spontaneous pain). Active MTPs are responsible for patient's pain. Local and referred pain from latent MTPs are not recognized by the patients; thus latent MTPs are not responsible for patient's pain.

Mechanisms of local pain and tenderness

Pressure pain threshold (PPT) measurement over an entire muscle shows the heterogeneous distribution (ie the sites with the lowest PPT corresponding to the locations of MTPs in healthy subjects), fibromyalgia and chronic tension type headache, indicating that muscle nociceptors are sensitized at MTPs. The sensitized nociceptors lead to an increased excitability of the nociceptive nerve ending. In addition to the nociceptor sensitization, non-nociceptors (mainly the large diameter muscle afferents) are also sensitized at MTPs; the non-nociceptors which normally do not contribute to pain perception are now involved in pain generation at MTPs. Thus, local pain and tenderness at MTPs are largely due to nociceptor sensitization with a lesser contribution from non-nociceptor sensitization.

Nociceptors and non-nociceptors sensitization at MTPs is a localized event in the muscle. The algesic substances are significantly increased at active MTP compared with latent MTP and normal muscle point. These algesic substances may partly be released from the peripheral sensitized nociceptors that drive the pain associated with tissue injury and may also be released from the sustained muscle fiber contraction within muscle taut band. A further study on both intramuscular and surface EMG activity recorded from an MTP for minutes revealed that the SEA was similar to a muscle cramp potential and that the increase in local muscle pain intensity was positively associated with the duration and amplitude of muscle cramp episodes. The firing frequency of motor units (14.5 ± 5.1 pulses per second) during electrically-induced muscle cramp is similar to that of the endplate spikes of the SEA in humans. Localized muscle cramps may induce intramuscular hypoxia, increased concentrations of algesic substances and direct mechanical stimulation of nociceptors and pain. Human experimental studies showed that the irritability of a MTP was highly correlated with the prevalence of the SEA in the MTP as lower PPTs were associated with higher amplitude of the SEA. An increased MTP sensitivity is associated with the occurrence of muscle cramps, and, glutamate injection into a latent MTP also increases sympathetic activity with a decreased blood supply to the muscle and the skin.

Thus, MTP pain and tenderness is closely associated with sustained focal ischemia and focal muscle contraction and/or cramps within muscle taut band. Muscle cramps may partly underlie local and referred pain in chronic musculoskeletal pain syndromes associated with active MTPs.

Mechanisms of referred pain from MTP

Referred pain is defined as the pain the patient feels at a remote site away from the location of an MTP. Referred pain from active MTPs is sometimes the sole complaint of patients with pain. A typical example is that patient feels pain in the front shoulder only but the pain actually comes from an active MTP in the infraspinatus.

The occurrence of referred pain is dependent on the sensitivity of an MTP. Active MTPs induce larger referred pain area and higher pain intensity than latent MTPs. Experimental human pain studies also showed that the maintenance of referred pain was dependent on ongoing nociceptive input from the site of primary muscle pain. Animal studies showed that sustained muscle damage might sensitize dorsal horn neurons and open silent synapses in adjacent segments and excite neurons that supplied the body regions in which the referred pain was felt. Sustained focal ischemia and the increased algesic substances associated with muscle contraction and/or muscle cramps at MTP may sensitize the dorsal horn neurons and supraspinal structures inducing referred pain. Referred pain is a reversible process of central sensitization or neuroplasticity maintained by increased peripheral nociceptive input from MTP. Inactivation of active MTP results in the disappearance of referred pain. It is important to note that referred pain usually occurs seconds following mechanical stimulation of an active MTP in humans, suggesting that the induction of neuroplastic changes related to referred pain is a very rapid process, similar to the induction of central descending inhibition mechanism which is recruited a few milliseconds following intramuscular nociceptive electrical stimulation.

Muscle taut band

An MTP taut band is subjectively felt by the examiner during manual palpation. Penetration of a needle into the taut band reveals a feeling of higher resistance as compared to surrounding normal muscle tissues by the practitioners. The existence of a taut band is demonstrated by magnetic resonance elastography, indicating that the stiffness of the taut bands may be 50% greater than that of the surrounding muscle tissue. Ultrasound visualization of the taut band show that MTPs appear as focal, hypoechoic regions on two-dimensional ultrasound and as focal regions of reduced vibration amplitude on vibration sonoelastography, indicating a localized, stiff nodule. These findings suggest that taut bands associated with MTP are detectable and quantifiable tools for MTP diagnosis.

The mechanisms for the formation of muscle taut band are not fully understood. The molecular mechanisms of taut band formation have been detailed in a recent review. SEA originates from the extrafusal motor endplate (motor unit potential) and the SEA represents focal muscle fiber contraction and/or muscle cramp. Muscle fiber contraction contributes significantly to the formation of muscle tension. It is believed that this involuntary focal muscle fiber contraction and/or muscle cramps within taut muscle band contributes significantly to muscle tension and to the formation of taut band associated with MTP Additional contributions to the formation of taut band may come from muscle spindle afferents giving afferent signals to the extrafusal motor unit through the H-reflex pathway and from the sympathetic facilitation to the SEA and to MTP sensitivity. Sympathetic neurotransmitter nor adrenaline not only strengthens muscle tone by boosting endogenous glutamate-mediated excitation, but also transforms sub-threshold glutamatergic activity into a robust excitatory drive capable of triggering motoneurone activity.

Thus, muscle taut band associated with MTP may come from increased motor unit excitability with an increased release of Ach and modulated by muscle spindle afferents and sympathetic hyperactivity. One of the peripheral pain generators in the muscle, MTP may have generalized effects on the human nociceptive system.

Role of MTPs in the Transition from Localized Pain to Generalized Pain Conditions

Apart from localized pain conditions, such as chronic tension type headache and migraine, myofascial low back pain, chronic prostatitis/chronic pelvic pain syndrome in men, lateral epicondylalgia, headache and mechanical neck pain and temporomandibular pain disorders, active MTPs contribute significantly to the generalized pain conditions, such as whiplash syndrome and fibromyalgia, suggesting that active MTPs play a significant role in the transition from the localized pain to generalized pain conditions. There are several ways whereby active MTPs may induce widespread pain or spatial pain propagation.

Active MTPs induce central sensitization

Central sensitization mechanisms are involved in both the localized and generalized chronic pain conditions. Descending facilitatory and inhibitory mechanisms are involved in acute muscle nociception. Persistent pain from tissue injury or inflammation contributes significantly to the induction of central sensitization and results in an enhanced net descending facilitation that contributes to the amplification and spread of pain. Mechanical stimulation or activation of latent MTPs induces mechanical hyperalgesia in extra segmental deep tissues and electrical stimulation of active MTPs significantly enhances somatosensory and limbic activity in the brain. Inactivation of active MTPs with consecutive anesthetic injections significantly decreases mechanical hyperalgesia and/or allodynia and referred pain in both localized pain condition of migraine and generalized pain conditions of fibromyalgia and whiplash syndrome. Thus, active MTPs are one of the sources of peripheral nociceptive input inducing central sensitization.

Central sensitization may increase the MTP sensitivity through segmental pathways resulting in decreased mechanical pain threshold and increased amplitude of the SEA. The influence of a central MTP on satellite MTPs may play a significant role in the segmental pain propagation in chronic generalized pain conditions; however, no evidence supports that central sensitization can induce the development of new MTPs. Further studies are needed to investigate the relationship between central sensitization and the MTP formation.

Active MTPs impair descending inhibition

In chronic musculoskeletal pain conditions, the balance between supraspinal facilitation and inhibition of pain shifts towards an overall decrease in inhibition. Muscle pain impairs diffuse noxious inhibitory control mechanisms. Inactivation of active MTPs with ultrasound and dry needling temporarily increases mechanical pain threshold in local pain syndromes. Inactivation of active MTPs results in an increased mechanical pain threshold in fibromyalgia patients. Active MTPs are one of the major contributors to the impaired descending inhibition in chronic musculoskeletal pain conditions. Impaired descending inhibition in chronic musculoskeletal pain conditions, which is same as an enhanced central sensitization, leads to an increased mechanical pain sensitivity of muscle tissue (ie muscle becomes more tender upon mechanical stimulation). Related to this mechanism, PPT at latent MTPs located in various body parts may become lower; latent MTPs are easily activated in response to various perpetuating factors. Pain propagation may thus be observed in the segmental and/or extrasegmental muscles in generalized chronic pain conditions.

Active MTPs impair motor control strategy

Upper trapezius muscle is active across the duration of shoulder activities and the frequency of differential activation between cranial and caudal regions within the upper trapezius is lower in fibromyalgia patients than controls. Sustained muscle activation induces muscle ischemia and increases the release of algesic substances in the muscle and cytokines in the blood and eventually decreases the muscle mechanical pain threshold more in the cranial region than the caudal region. Sustained muscle contraction at low load levels may damage muscle tissues and increase MTP sensitivity and latent MTPs may be activated and result in local and referred pain. An increased muscle co-activation has also been observed in local pain conditions, such as tension type headache. An increased co-activation of antagonist musculature may reflect reorganization of the motor control strategy in patients, potentially leading to muscle overload and increased nociception. While active MTPs are present in these patients, there is no direct evidence on whether the impaired motor control strategy is associated with the existence of active MTPs. However, latent MTPs are associated with impaired motor activation pattern and the elimination of these latent MTPs induces normalization of the impaired motor activation pattern. The impaired motor control strategy may partially underlie the induction of local pain and segmental pain propagation.

Local compression by taut bands (muscle fibers that shorten in the absence of propagating action potentials) can impair arterial inflow and reduce the supply of oxygen, calcium, and other nutrients necessary for energy-dependent muscle relaxation and higher energy demands required by the aberrantly sustained muscle contraction. Continued, persistent sarcomere contractures can distort and damage involved tissues, which may precipitate the synthesis and release of endogenous algogenic biochemicals and inflammatory substances that enhance nociception. These effects suggest that persistent or chronic pain perception associated with MPS can involve numerous proinflammatory cytokines, neurotransmitters, and neuromodulators, including tumor necrosis factor- (TNF-), substance P, and cyclooxygenase-2 (COX-2), which relay pain signals from the peripheral to the central nervous system. An increase in -endorphin level can suppress neurons from releasing substance P and thus, inhibit pain transmission. These observations, which provide biochemical evidence, correlated with recent, partially approved studies that demonstrated significantly higher concentrations of substance P and TNF- in the local surroundings of active MTrPs. Moreover, a number of hypoxc-responsive proteins, including hypoxia-inducible factor-1, vascular endothelial growth factor (VEGF), and stimulate isoform of nitric oxide synthases (iNOS), can be found in response to hypoxia and mechanical stimulation in skeletal muscles.

Classification of the Trigger Points

The critical part of evaluation of the skeletal muscle is finding the location of trigger points and understanding their nature. Let's start with the definition of the trigger point. Despite the fact that the patient feels the trigger point as a pain with a pin-point location, the area of the muscle which carries the trigger point isn't in a round form, but can be best described as having a spindle- like form within the muscle tissue. Thus, trigger point is a part of the hypertonus where a number of the muscular fibers exhibit the strongest spasm. This spasm is a fundamental cause of trigger point formation because it diminishes blood circulation through the affected tissues (Fassbender, Wegner, 1973; Popelansky et al., 1976; Travell, Simons, 1983, etc.).

According to the world wide accepted classification (Travel and Simmons, 1983) the trigger points in the skeletal muscles separated on:

- Active trigger point (ATP)
- Latent or "sleeping" trigger point (LTP)
- Satellite or referred trigger point (STP)
- Secondary trigger points (SCTP)
- Motor trigger point (MTP)

1. **Active trigger point (ATP)**

   The ATP(s) hold the key to the muscle tension and pain in the affected area. ATP is the area of the greatest pain felt by the patient during active movements or while the practitioner applies direct pressure on it. The ATP forced the patient to start looking for help. This trigger point is an epicenter of acute pain. The pain from the ATP usually radiates along the fibers of the same muscle or along the entire muscle group. Another important symptom to remember is muscle weakness. A muscle with ATP becomes weak to the degree of being unable to execute motor commands from the central nervous system. ATP in every skeletal muscle has the tendency to form in the same areas. This is why the map of trigger points is a helpful diagnostic tool.

2. **Latent or "sleeping" trigger point (LTP)**

   LTP is an active trigger point which, as a result of self-treatment or inappropriate professional treatment, was not eliminated but transferred into a so-called "sleeping" state. The LTP does not bother the patient either during physical activity or during the rest, but is the major cause of stiffness (especially in the morning). Muscles which harbor LTPs are easily fatigued, and weaker. LTPs may also trigger moderate pain at the very end of movement. LTP can be easily reactivated and become active ones and vice versa. In a sense, the LTP is the chronic presence of the condition of hyperirritability of the muscle spindle receptors. Thus, reactivation of the LTP can be caused by any factor, from physical overload to changes in the surrounding temperature. The constant transition of the active trigger point into the latent state and back is the major cause of the formation of the core of myogelosis.

3. **Satellite or referred trigger point (STP)**

   STP is also painful areas of muscular tension. However, the intensity of the pain is less and they are smaller. STPs also contribute to the overall muscular weakness, pain, and tension. The patient does not feel STPs the same as he or she feels active ones. They are mostly felt as a radiation of the pain from the active trigger point (Jacobs, 1960; Popelansky, et all, 1976; Travell, Simmons, 1983). Thus, to detect the location of the STP, the practitioner has to ask the patient about the patterns of the pain radiation from the active trigger point, and examine these areas.

4. **Secondary trigger points (SCTP)**

   All muscles which are responsible for movement in the joint are separated into "prime movers" and "synergists". A prime mover is the muscle mostly responsible for this particular movement in the joint. Muscle synergist helps the prime mover when extra force is needed for the specific tasks. For example the prime mover of the elbow flexion is biceps brachii muscle, but synergists of the same movement are brachialis and brachioradialis muscles. SCTPs are formed in the muscles-synergists as a result of their overload. If biceps brachii harbors an active trigger point it becomes weaker and it is unable to provide all the necessary force for the flexion of the elbow on its own. In such a case, the brachialis and brachioradialis muscles start to work harder. However, they were not designed to be prime movers. Both muscles are supposed to work only as assistants. Now they have to participate in every flexion of the elbow. As a result of their overload, secondary trigger points start to develop.

5. **Motor trigger point (MTP)**

   MTPs are located in the areas of neuro-muscular junction where the motor nerve which innervates the muscle enters it. Several studies on the subject of MTPs showed that in these areas the strongest muscular contractions are registered if the weakest electric current was applied. Usually MTP are secondary reaction to the nerve irritation or chronic muscle and fascia tension. According to histologically conducted studies (Heine, 1997; Gogoleva, 2001) chronic pain and low grade tension in the skeletal muscles and fascia are responsible for the low grade inflammation around the terminal parts of motor nerve which ends at the neuro-muscular junction. This chronic inflammation activates the local fibroblasts, which deposit collagen around the nerve endings forming so-called "collagen cuffs". These "collagen cuffs" detected around the neuro-muscular junctions interfere with very intimate neurochemical process of transferring impulse from the nerve tissue to the muscle tissue. This mechanism is responsible for the generation of pain in the area of MTP(s). MTPs have very unique diagnostic value. According to several studies, the abundant presence of motor trigger points is a sign of spinal nerve irritation or compression by the bulging disk or other structures in the area of the vertebral segment (Gunn et all, 1976).

EVALUATION OF THE TRIGGER POINTS IN THE SKELETAL MUSCLES

There are several types of the trigger points in the skeletal muscles. In very complicated, chronic cases of the long existing muscle pathology several types of the trigger points may co-exists at the same time and this is the most confusing part of TrP.

Evaluation of Active Trigger Points (ATP)

ATP is the most painful symptom of the muscle tension. It is critically important to detect the ATP at the very beginning. It is relatively simple task if the patient has fresh case and ATP is single. The situation becomes much more difficult if the practitioner deals with the chronic muscle pathology. In such case the satellite, secondary or motor trigger points further complicates the examination process and frequently mislead the practitioner.

The earliest detection of the ATP is a must because it frequently holds the key to entire tension in the affected area. If the practitioner made incorrect decision and addressed secondary trigger point instead of the ATP he or she fights with windmills.

Steps for diagnosing:

- **Questioning**

  Ask the patient to pinpoint the most painful area and after this ask him or her to show the movement which triggers the most intense pain in this area. Match this information with the map of trigger points.

- **Palpation**

  Palpation is as much an art as it is a science. Patient must be relaxed sufficiently to gain access to vulnerable and potentially painful treatment. A thorough case history and directed questioning is essential. It is important to talk to the patient and explain the procedure to reduce the patient's anxiety levels, and allows participation in the treatment process. Involving the patient is a key step, as feedback from the patient helps to locate the exact centre of the trigger point.

  Technique
  - Finger pads palpation: remember to cut your finger nails (shorter is better);
  - Flat palpation: use the fingertips to slide around the patient's skin across muscle fibers;
  - Pincer palpation: pinch the belly of the muscle between the thumb and the other fingers, rolling muscle fibers back and forth;
  - Flat hand palpation: useful in the abdominal region (viscera);
  - Elbow: allows stronger leverage which can be an advantage.
  - Algometer can be used for measuring point tenderness and pain generated by pressure.

  Findings:
  - Stiffness in the affected muscle;
  - Spot tenderness (exquisite pain);
  - A palpable taut nodule or band;
  - Presence of referred pair;
  - Reproduction of the patient's symptoms (accurate);
  - May be hotter (or colder) than the surrounding tissues;
  - May be more moist than the surrounding tissues;
  - May feel a little like sand paper;
  - May be a loss of skin elasticity in the region of the trigger point.

- **"Jump Symptom" Test**

  There is a limited number of diagnostic tools to evaluate hypertonic muscular abnormalities and the "Jump Symptom" is still the most effective one (Fisher, 1988). Always start with palpation of the affected area using pressure just below the threshold of pain. Try to detect structural changes (e.g., dense areas, tight bands, etc.) within the examined muscle. Ask the patient to report any pain sensations and their intensity during the examination. After this, apply pressure above the threshold of pain in the suspected areas.

  If the examiner hits a trigger point, the patient will feel acute pain and react with the so called "jump symptom" which is withdrawal of the examined segment or entire body from the practitioner (Kraft, et all 1968).

- **Range of Motion test**

  If the patient has a new case of hypertonic muscular abnormality with one trigger point and one affected muscle, the diagnostic evaluation is an easy task. The situation becomes much more complicated when the hypertonic abnormality has a long history and there is a clinical picture of widespread pain and muscle tension. In such cases, the application of pressure on any area along the affected and neighboring muscles will produce the "Jump Symptom". However, as we discussed above, the ATP must be treated and eliminated first. It becomes impossible for the practitioner to differentiate between active trigger points and other TrP as each of them produces pain of the same intensity. The Movement Test is specially designed for these cases. It is very simple and informative.

Ask the patient to perform movement in the joint or part of the body which causes the pain. Now, press finger in the area being examined and ask the patient to repeat the same movement. If the practitioner presses into the ATP the patient will be able to repeat the same movements without pain or with a very tolerable amount of it as long as the practitioner maintains the compression of the tissue. As soon as the practitioner releases the finger and asks the patient to repeat the same movement, he or she will feel the pain again and stop movement as soon as the critical level of contraction is reached. In other words, the practitioner uses pressure to deactivate the ATP, and as long as it is deactivated, the muscle is able to productively contract.

If the practitioner examines the satellite trigger point instead of the ATP the patient will still have pain in the tested muscle during its contraction despite the fact that the practitioner is maintaining the compression of soft tissue. Thus, the Movement Test allows to differentiate between various types of trigger points and to find the active one quickly.

- **Evaluation of Latent Trigger Points (LTP)**
  The patient who has LTP never complains about pain or uncomfortable sensations in the affected area. The most he or she will mention is morning stiffness which usually disappears in hour or two. The only way the practitioner may detect the LTP is a "Jump Symptom" Test. If the practitioner applies pressure in the LTP the patient exhibits classical reaction of body withdrawal and this pain disappears as soon as the pressure discontinues. Usually the clients very surprise to feel pain in these areas because they never bothered them. If LTP present this area(s) must be included into the treatment protocol and LTP should go through the same therapy as ATP.

- **Evaluation of Satellite Trigger Points (STP)**
  STP is easy to find as soon as practitioner determines the ATP. The practitioner should ask the patient about any pain radiation. If the pain radiates to the distant areas, for example ATP in the pectoralis major muscle accompanies by the radiation of the pain to the hand, the practitioner can be sure that he or she deals with the radiation of the pain along the peripheral nerve. However if the patient complains about radiation of the pain from the anterior surface of the shoulder joint to the anterior chest the practitioner can be sure that this pathway of the pain radiation is associated with the ATP in the pectoralis major muscle.
  The best way to examine muscle for the presence of STP is to apply pressure along the pathway of the pain radiation which patient showed during questioning. Usually during the application of pressure the patient does not exhibit classic jump sign because intensity of the pain is much less in the STP(s). Also, remember or record the location of STP because they need to be completely deactivated during the treatment.

- **Evaluation of the Secondary Trigger points (SCTP)**
  SCTP is much more rare compare to all other types of the trigger points. Usually they formed when long lasting chronic muscle tension is present in the prime movers. The palpation of muscle synergists is the only way to detect tension there. The only problem with the muscle synergists is, that they are frequently located under the e prime movers. Thus to examine the muscle synergists the practitioner should be familiar with approach to mobilize the superficially located prime mover to get to the muscle-synergist directly without eliciting pressure on the superficially located muscle.

Criteria for Identifying a Latent Trigger Point or an Active Trigger Point

- **Essential Criteria**
  - Palpable taut band (if muscle accessible).
  - Exquisite spot tenderness of a nodule in a taut band.
  - Patient's recognition of current pain complaint by pressure on the tender nodule,
  - Painful limit to full stretch range of motion.
- **Confirmatory Observations**
  - Visual or tactile identification of local twitch response.

- o Local twitch response induced by needle penetration of tender nodule.
- o Pain or altered sensation (in the distribution expected from a trigger point in that muscle) on compression of tender nodule.
- o Electromyographic demonstration of spontaneous electrical activity characteristic of active loci in the tender nodule of a taut band.

Causes of Trigger Points

Understanding what causes trigger points to occur and reoccur in the body's muscles is absolutely critical to achieving a successful treatment. Therapist become too focused on finding and releasing active trigger points, and give little thought as to what caused the trigger points to occur in the first place. Such a superficial approach is doomed to always be one step behind in treatment of myofascial pain disorders. Success depends on understanding what causes trigger points to develop in muscles and then asking the right questions.

The Primary Cause of Trigger Points is Muscular Overload

To most people, the term muscular overload probably conjures up images of physical strain on the muscle tissue and its tendons, but in trigger point therapy the term has a dual interpretation. While the physical load imposed on a muscle does play a role in trigger point formation, an equally important factor is the demand placed on the neuromuscular control mechanism of the muscle. This mechanism is responsible for taking the electrical impulse of a nerve and transforming it into a biochemical signal that both controls and powers muscular activity. The complex nature of this electrochemical process makes it the "weak link in the chain" of muscular functioning, and the failure of a muscle's control mechanism is responsible for the activation of trigger points.

Understanding the different types of muscular overload.

Muscular overload comes in several different ways; some are obvious, while others are a bit more elusive. Let's take a closer look at each type of muscular overload:

- **Exertion Overload:** This is the most obvious form of muscular overload and simply means that a muscle was not strong enough to perform a task required of it. For example, bending at the waist to lift a heavy object is likely to create an exertion overload in the low back muscles. Trigger point activity resulting from this type of overload is more prominent in unconditioned muscles. People who take part in resistance training (lifting weights) are likely to develop exertion related trigger points when they just begin training, or return to it after a long hiatus. Most of the time, this type of overload occurs in a sudden fall, when a person tries to brace against an impact.
- **Overuse or Repetitive Stress Overload:** An overload of this type is probably the most common cause of trigger point activity. In these cases, the muscle's functional endurance is exceeded by a given task. Examples include performing repetitive movements at a job day after day, sporting activities, and gardening.
- **Biomechanical Overload:** Muscles work together in functional groupings called myotatic units to create bodily movement. For any given movement, the muscles within a myotatic unit can be classified into two groups: synergists and antagonists. Synergistic muscles work together to produce a specific bodily movement, while antagonistic muscles act to produce the opposing bodily movement. Biomechanical overload occurs when one of the muscles in a myotatic unit is weakened by trigger point activity. In this situation, a synergistic muscle becomes overloaded by the additional work load that it must take on because of its dysfunctional partner, and an antagonistic muscle becomes overloaded by a distortion in the nerve supply controlling it. Trigger point formation in a muscle due to biomechanical overload occurs frequently in established myofascial pain disorders, and must be recognized to treat these disorders effectively
- **Postural Overload:** One of the more subtle ways of overloading a muscle is to place it in an over-shortened or overstretched state for a prolonged period of time. This type of overload, termed postural overload, can be either of a mechanical or neurological nature, and is closely related to biomechanical overload. There are two very common types of postural overload that cause trigger points to form within a muscle; antalgic and degenerative. Antalgic postural overloads occur when a person holds their body in a certain manner to avoid the pain from an injury. For example, a person may hold their head to one side to diminish the

pain from a neck cramp, or lean their trunk forward to avoid aggravating a backache. Degenerative postural overloads occur secondarily to the long-term changes in posture associated with aging or disease. Examples include an exaggerated sway in the lower back, or the forward head and sunken chest posture so frequently seen in older adults. In either type of postural overload, some muscles are kept in abnormally shortened position, while others are kept in an abnormally elongated position, predisposing both groups of muscles to the development of trigger points.

- **Referred Pain Overload:** Pain that is referred to a muscle from trigger points in other muscles, or from joints and internal organs, can overload a muscle's control mechanism and cause trigger points to form within it. In trigger point therapy, trigger points that develop secondarily to the referred pain from other trigger points are called satellite trigger points. Any myofascial disorder that is more than 2 days old, is likely to involve satellite trigger point activity. If the referred pain is severe enough, muscle tension associated with an unconscious guarding reflex may also produce trigger point activity in the local muscles.

- **Muscle Trauma Overload:** Physical trauma to a muscle, like that which might occur during a fall or automobile accident, can directly activate trigger points in that muscle. This may occur from a reflex response to the pain associated with the tissue damage, or because of impairment in the muscle's functional capacity.

Factors That Predispose a Muscle to Overload

The following is a list of factors that can make a muscle particularly susceptible to the types of muscular overload discussed above. In cases where trigger point activity returns shortly after treatment, one should investigate these conditions for a likely cause.

- **Muscle Tension:** Anything that increases a muscle's tension also makes it more susceptible to muscular overload. Emotional stress can create significant tension in the neck, shoulder, and abdominal muscles, making these muscles hot-spots of trigger point activity. One frequently overlooked source of muscular tension results from chilling the muscle, like that which might occur when sleeping under a ceiling fan. Some neurological disorders, like strokes, can cause abnormalities in muscle tension as well.

- **Structural Inadequacies:** This term refers to abnormalities in the skeletal structure that can cause some muscles to be chronically overworked when trying to compensate for them. Examples include having one leg that is longer than the other (a lower limb-length inequality), pelvic bone asymmetries, short upper arms, and a Morton foot structure (short big toe-long second toe).

- **Nutritional Deficiencies:** Myofascial pain disorders can be perpetuated by deficiencies in the water-soluble vitamins B1, B6, B12, folic acid, and vitamin C. These micronutrients play important roles in the physiology of muscular activity and nearly half of chronic myofascial pain disorder cases require dietary supplementation for successful treatment. Additionally, dietary imbalances in calcium, potassium, and iron may also perpetuate trigger point disorders, and must be corrected to achieve long-term treatment success in some cases.

- **Metabolic Disorders:** Any abnormality in the energy metabolism of a muscle can make it hypersensitive to overload stress. Systemic metabolic disorders such as hypothyroidism and hypoglycemia can contribute significantly to the perpetuation of trigger point activity in muscles throughout the body.

- **Chronic Bacterial Infections:** Dental abscesses, sinusitis, and urinary tract infections may negate the treatment of trigger points, and must be ruled out in relevant cases.

- **Viral Diseases:** Systemic viral conditions such as the flu or herpes simplex virus 1 (not genital herpes) need to be addressed prior to the treatment of trigger point disorders.

CHAPTER 2- UNDERSTANDING DRY NEEDLING

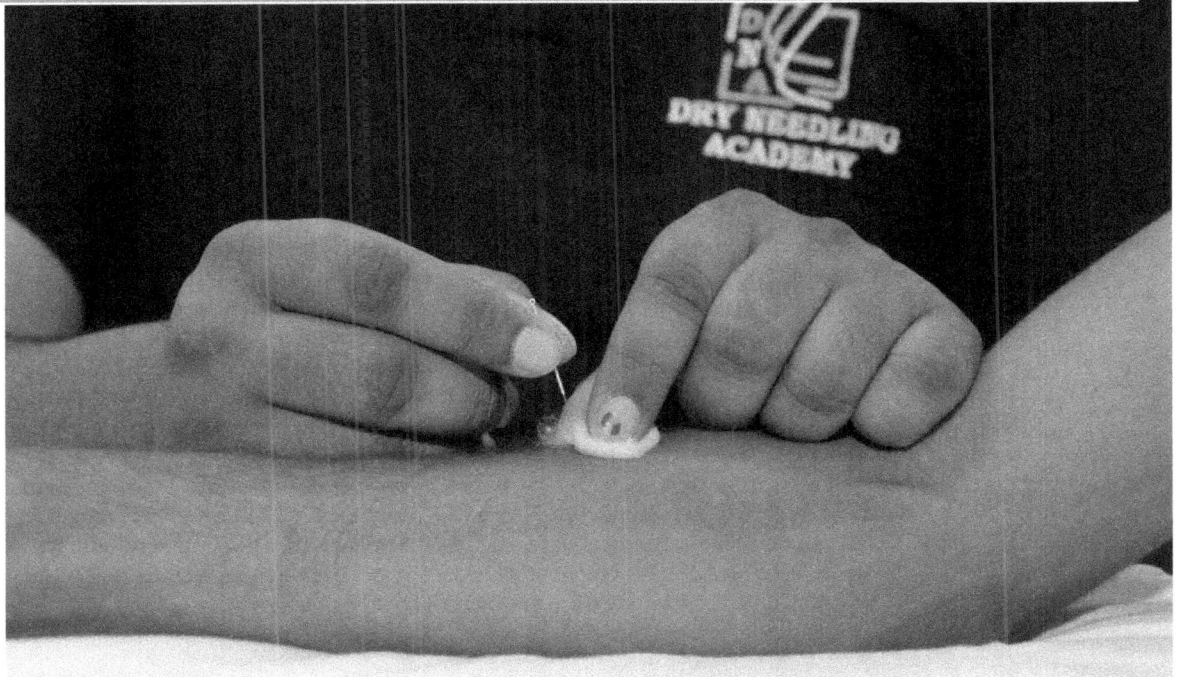

DRY NEEDLING TECHNIQUE

Models of Dry Needling

The dry needling techniques have possessed many perspective while its evolution since its came into picture. Some of the models used by different therapist in incorporating dry needling as a treatment tool are discussed below:

The 4 models are as following:
1. The Radiculopathy Model,
2. The Trigger Point Model,
3. The Spinal Segmental Sensitization and Pentad Model.

- **The Radiculopathy Model**

  This model, proposed by C.C. Gunn, states that the myofascial pain syndromes (MPS) are always the result of peripheral neuropathy. He defines peripheral neuropathy as 'a condition that causes disordered function in the peripheral nerve'. (The peripheral nerve exists after the nerve leaves the spinal column). Gunn considers spondylosis, or bony/spur formation, as the most likely cause. He also discussed how the deep spinal tissues and muscles, such as the multifidi, can lead to disc compression or intervertebral foramina (hole where nerve comes out from spinal cord) compression and irritation. This irritation causes nerve irritation, and this causes neuropathy, thus supporting his model.

  Simply stated, Gunn believes that tender points and trigger points in the body are a result of spinal nerve dysfunction and many times are not as a result of a problem at the local level. This model parallels a lot of what is taught to chiropractic students as the neurological system affects all functions of the body. Sensitized nerves can lead to soft tissue compromise as the nerves determine the health of the body and the nerves start at the spinal cord. Striated muscle, which accounts for 40 percent of total body mass, is then adversely impacted by impaired neurological function, and this leads to tender points and dysfunctional soft tissue.

  Due to these facts, Gunn's treatment is aimed at the musculo-tendinous (where muscle becomes tendon) junction, or the location of the muscle motor points, because this is where the muscle is most likely innervated by the nerves. So, he treated the area where he identified tender points/trigger points. In addition, the spinal level associated with this region must be treated as the small local nerves, which innervate the multifidi and other associated spinal structures, will have pathology that needs to be addressed. It is important to note that unless the proximal spinal level is treated (assuming there is dysfunction at the spinal level), the distal component will not resolve. To better understand this, it is important to point out that the nerves in the paraspinal muscles as well as at the associated distal locations is linked and this is why it is necessary to treat both.

- **The Trigger Point Model**

  Myofascial Trigger Points (MTrPs, or TrPs for Trigger Points) are defined as 'hyper-irritable spots in skeletal muscle that are associated with a hypersensitive palpable nodule in a taut band' (Travell and Simons). The resultant pain/discomfort that one gets due to such points is referred to as myofascial pain syndrome (MPS). Simply, MPS is defined as 'sensory, motor, and autonomic symptoms caused by myofascial trigger points' (Travell and Simons). Sensory symptoms refer to what one feel, motor symptoms refer to how the muscles work, and autonomic symptoms refer to the things that one does not realize. This seems a little odd, but considers what happens when one bang his arm really hard. He will feel the pain (sensory), the muscle might be painful and not contract properly (motor), and his heart rate goes up as does his respiration, due to the 'adrenaline rush' (autonomic) of the injury.

  MTrPs exist where there is macro (large) trauma and/or micro (small or repetitive use injury) trauma. These traumas cause an excessive release of calcium in the muscle and this leads to shortening of the muscle. When the damage goes untreated, the excessive shortening begins to cut off oxygen supply to the area, adversely affecting the cell's ability to produce

ATP. Without ATP, the muscle cannot relax. To go along with this, excessive acetylcholine (a neurotransmitter responsible for activating muscles) release is found in the areas of MTrPs. Along with the lack of ATP, the excessive acetylcholine helps to form the knotted, tight/taut muscle fibers associated with MTrPs. The acetylcholine cannot be broken down due to the altered function and toxic state in the MTrP. In effect, the toxicity is due the acidic environment and this acidity inhibits the breakdown of the acetylcholine. To top it all off, the area will also have a lot of byproducts of pathological muscle function such as serotonin, leukotrienes, prostaglandins, bradykinins, and more. These byproducts further the inflammatory and pathological state of the tissue, causing pain and dysfunction.

There are 2 most common types of MTrPs (but there are four types that are discussed later):
1. Active TrPs that cause pain in the location of the actual TrP and refer pain or altered sensation (paresthesia) distally.
2. Latent TrPs, which do the same thing, but they must first be stimulated to do so.

So, with the TrPs model, taut bands, very tender spots on the band, a 'jump' sign (pain catches so quickly that it makes the body jerk), and pain recognition are typically found if a skilled manual therapist is applying the dry needling. It is interesting to note that trigger points, if active or latent, tend to show up in the same parts of the particular muscle(s) on everyone. So, a TrP found in the vastus lateralis muscle (lateral quadriceps muscle) on one person, if he/she has TrPs in that muscle; will tend to show up in the same place/places of the vastus lateralis on another person, if that person also has TrPs in that muscle.

Dry needling is used to help diagnose and treat TrPs and it can be used to elicit the The Local Twitch Response (LTR). This is really the basic and essential aspect of dry needling according to the Trigger Point Model. The LTR is an involuntary spinal cord reflex contraction of the muscle fibers in a tight/taut band following treatment or needling of the band/TrP. According to the TrP model, when applying a deep type of therapy, such as dry needling, eliciting the LTR is necessary. In effect, the LTR confirms that the needle was put in the right place, and by doing so, likely resolution of the trigger point is achieved. This, in turns, help to eliminate pain and dysfunction in the area being treated.

- **Spinal Segmental Sensitization and Pentad Model**
  The Spinal Segmental Sensitization (SSS) and Pentad Model was proposed by the late Andrew Fischer, M.D. (Physiatrist, pain management and rehabilitation medical doctor). This is a good time to discuss this model as it really incorporates both of the first two models. Dr. Fischer proposed that the SSS is a 'hyperactive' state of the dorsal horn of the spinal cord that is caused by damaged tissue sending nociceptive (pain) input into the spinal cord. This information then causes the over-sensitivity of the associated spinal level dermatome (skin), pain sensitivity of the associated spinal level sclerotome (bone, ligaments, joints), and Myofascial Trigger Points (MTrPs) in the associated spinal level muscles. All this occurs because the nerve coming from the spine is over sensitized, and by being in this pathological state, it stimulates these changes listed above. In effect, there is a vicious cycle of pain and dysfunction.

  It is important to note that MTrPs in the spinal level associated musculature and tender spots in the supraspinous and interspinous ligaments of the spine of the associated level can lead to SSS due to their nociceptive bombardment. What matters most here is that the damaged tissue is bombarding the spinal cord (dorsal horn, in particular) with pain input. All of this pain and neurological irritation eventually trigger a response at the anterior horn of the spinal cord. The anterior horn is responsible for muscle function along the spinal level and when the anterior horn is sending out improper information to the muscle(s), MTrPs can form. (It's like information from the body goes into the dorsal horn of the spinal cord, it is then processed and information from the spinal cord out goes through the anterior horn), all of this leads to dysfunction and pain. With this model, like Gunn's Radiculopathy Model, the spinal level problem affects the distal associated skin, muscles, and ligaments/joints.

So, treatment must be applied to the spinal area to shut off the stimuli from the supraspinous and interspinous ligaments so that the dorsal horn is not activated. There is no better way to get to spinal ligaments than with dry needling. If the dorsal horn gets activated, then there will be carryover to the anterior horn, and the body will be affected. With the SSS treatment approach, treating the MTrPs can shut off the afferent (going towards the spinal cord) stimuli. In effect, the entire vicious cycle must be stopped. This model is very big into identifying the spinal region of dysfunction as addressing the proximal problem should clear out the distal one(s).

Dr. Fischer balanced the information from the Gunn and Travell models. He values the treatment of the peripheral problems, but treating the spinal location is of utmost importance. Dry needling allows the trained practitioner to treat the spinal level of a problem as well as the distal problem. One of the main objectives of dry needling is to identify and destroy MTrPs. In addition, as per the SSS model, unless one administer a technique such as dry needling, it is virtually impossible to address the interspinous and supraspinous ligaments.

Fischer's Pentad Model is a set of 5 signs that go together to support the SSS. They are:
1. Supraspinous ligament sprain,
2. Radicular involvement from the spinal level problem,
3. Segmental paraspinal muscle spasm,
4. Narrowed space between the spinous processes,
5. Narrowed disc and IVF spaces that lead to additional stress that injures, or sprains, the interspinous and supraspinous ligaments.

Type of Dry Needling Procedures

Dry needling is commonly used to deactivate and treat myofascial trigger points. Effectiveness of dry needling in the management of MTrPs has been evaluated in numerous RCTs and systematic reviews. The recent Cochrane systematic review of 35 RCTs, 23 assessed the efficacy of dry needling for management of low back pain. It was concluded that there is evidence of pain relief and functional improvement of chronic low back pain with the use of dry needling compared with no treatment or sham therapy.

As per the site and depth of needle penetration used to treat a myofascial trigger point, dry needling procedures are categorized into:
- Superficial Dry needling,
- Deep Dry Needling.

Superficial Dry Needling

In the early 1980s, Baldry was concerned about the risk of causing a pneumothorax when treating a patient with an MTrP in the anterior scalene muscle. Rather than using TrP-DDN, he inserted the needle superficially into the tissue immediately overlying the MTrP. After leaving the needle in for a short time, the exquisite tenderness at the MTrP was abolished and the spontaneous pain was alleviated. Based on this experience, Baldry expanded the practice of SDN and applied the technique to MTrPs throughout the body with good empirical results, even in the treatment of MTrPs in deeper muscles. He recommended inserting a dry needle into the tissues overlying each MTrP to a depth of 5-10 mm for 30 seconds. Because the needle does not necessarily reach the MTrP, LTRs are not expected. Nevertheless, the patient commonly experiences an immediate decrease in sensitivity following the needling procedure. If there is any residual pain, the needle is reinserted for another 2-3 minutes. When using the TrP-SDN technique, Baldry commented that the amount of needle stimulation depends on an individual's responsiveness. In average responders, Baldry recommended leaving the needle in situ for 30-60 seconds. In weak responders, the needle may be left for up to 2 or 3 minutes. There is some evidence from animal studies that this responsiveness is at least partially genetically determined. Mice deficient in endogenous opioid peptide receptors did not respond well to needle-evoked nerve stimulation. Baldry suggested that weak responders might have excessive amounts of endogenous opioid peptide antagonists. Baldry preferred TrP-SDN over TrP-DDN, but indicated that in cases where MTrPs were secondary to the development of radiculopathy, he would consider using TrP-DDN.

Another SDN technique was developed in 1996 in China. Initially, Fu's subcutaneous needling (FSN), also referred to as "floating needling," was developed to treat various pain problems without consideration of MTrPs, such as chronic low back pain, fibromyalgia, osteoarthritis, chronic pelvic pain, post-herpetic pain, peripheral neuropathy, and complex regional pain syndrome. In a recent paper, Fu et al applied their needling technique to MTrPs and examined whether the direction of the needle is relevant in that treatment. The needle was either directed across muscle fibers or along muscle fibers toward an MTrP. The authors concluded that FSN had an immediate effect on inactivating MTrPs in the neck, irrespective of the direction of the needle. The FSN needle consists of three parts: a 31 mm beveled-tip needle with a 1 mm diameter, a soft tube similar to an intravenous catheter, and a cap. The needle is directed toward a painful spot or MTrP at an angle of $20–30^0$ with the skin but does not penetrate muscle tissue. The technique acts solely in the subcutaneous layers. The needle is advanced parallel to the skin surface until the soft tube is also under the skin. At that time, the needle is moved smoothly and rhythmically from side to side for at least two minutes, after which the needle is removed from the soft tube, which stays in place. Patients go home with the soft tube still inserted under the skin. The soft tube can move slightly underneath the skin because of patient's movements and is thought to continue to stimulate subcutaneous connective tissues while in place. The soft tube is kept under the skin for a few hours for acute injuries and for at least 24 hours for chronic pain problems, after which it is removed. According to Fu et al, the technique has no adverse or side effects and usually induces an immediate reduction of pain. The needle techniques were not painful as subcutaneous layers are poorly innervated. Because FSN was only recently introduced to the Western world, the technique has not been used much outside of China and there are no other clinical outcome studies.

Advantages of SDN

The reasons for advocating the use of SDN for those with primary nociceptive MTrP pain are as follows:

- From its successful use, in a very large number of patients with such pain, over a considerable number of years, there can be little or no doubt as to its effectiveness.
- The procedure is very easily carried out.
- In contrast to DDN it is a painless procedure other than for an initial short sharp prick.
- There is minimal risk of damage to nerves, blood vessels and other structures.
- Because of minimal bleeding there is a low incidence of post-treatment soreness.

Deep Dry Needling:

As discussed in introduction chapter

"Dry needling is a skilled intervention that uses a thin filiform needle to penetrate the skin and stimulate underlying myofascial trigger points, muscular, and connective tissues for the management of neuromusculoskeletal pain and movement impairments"

We will be discussing deep dry needling in detail in following chapter and its application techniques for upper and lower quarter muscles.

Physiological Effects of Dry Needling
(1) Analgesic Effects

I.   Segmental Analgesia

The needles stimulate small myelinated ('Aδ') nerves in muscle and skin; these activate the small intermediate cells n the dorsal horn, by way of collateral terminals. The intermediate cells release the neuromodulator enkephalin, which blocks the transmission of pain in the substantia gelatinosa cells, and part of the nociceptive pathway (from the unmyelinated C fibres). The effect of enkephalin can be detected as a generalized depression of activity of the dorsal horn (Sandkuhler 2000). The effect is known as 'segmental analgesia', and takes some minutes to develop, but then outlasts the duration of the dry needling stimulation, possibly even lasting several days.

Segmental analgesia is inhibition of the nociceptive pathway at approximately the same spinal level in the dorsal horn.

II. Neuromodulators: opioid peptides

Dry needling has shown to release naturally occurring opioid peptides. Four opioid peptides have now been identified, but their complete roles in pain perception are still not fully understood. Each peptide is predominant in a different area of the CNS: β-endorphin is found in the brain and enkephalin in the spinal cord, and dry needling causes both to be released. Dynorphin, in the spinal cord and brainstem, has variable effects depending on the circumstances. Orphanin (also known as endomorphin or nociceptin) is widely distributed throughout forebrain, midbrain and spinal cord and has a multitude of functions in nociception, other sensory functions and autonomic control.

TABLE 1. Comparison of properties of the main opioid peptides

Peptide	Main site	Receptor	Blockage by naloxone	Relevant EA frequency (Hz)
β-endorphin	Midbrain, PAG (pituitary)	μ & δ	Low dose	Low (2–4)
Enkephalin	Dorsal horn of spinal cord	μ & δ	Low dose	Low (2–4)
Dynorphin	Brainstem and spine	K	High dose	High (50–100)
Orphanin	Widespread	M	Unknown	Low (2–4)

These opioid peptides are often referred to as neuromodulators rather than neurotransmitters, because, rather than producing a single response on one occasion only, they have a sustained effect and modify the activity of the target cell over a period of time. Three types of opioid receptor have been identified, called μ, δ and κ. These are not matched exactly to the different peptides, and some of the peptides stimulate more than one receptor. β-endorphin plays an important role in needling analgesia. In a piece of research that has become a landmark, needling increased the concentrations of β-endorphin in the CSF of patients with pain, whereas control group patients who did not receive dry needling showed no changes (Clement-Jones et al 1980). Subsequent studies have shown that the analgesic effect of dry needling has a slow onset, reaches a peak after about 20 minutes, and then decays slowly after removing the needles. This time pattern is entirely consistent with the action of neuromodulator release.

The evidence that opioid peptides are involved in needling has been reinforced by the discovery that some of the effects of needling can be reversed by naloxone, both in the laboratory (Han & Terenius 1982, Pomeranz & Chiu 1976) and in clinical trials in patients with pain (Mayer et al 1977). The discovery of specific antagonists to the different receptors has been crucially important in working out the roles of the different opioid peptides.

Knowledge of the central effects of DN upon opioid release is limited. Using functional magnetic resonance imaging, Niddam et al. [53] showed that pain following the insertion of a needle into a trigger point, combined with electrical stimulation, is mediated through the PAG in the brainstem. The PAG is a central part of the opioid circuitry that controls nociceptive transmission at the level of spinal cord and cortex. The change in PAG-activity was correlated with the change in PPT (pressure pain threshold). It is hypothesized that DN, via stimulation of the nociceptive fibers, may activate the enkephalinergic inhibitory dorsal horn interneurons. It is unclear whether the needle manipulation or the electrical stimulation is responsible for these results or both. This combination, being "electro-Dry needling", is also mentioned in clinical studies on dry needling-induced analgesia and laboratory results report endogenous opiate peptides to be involved.

III.   Non-opioid mechanisms in Dry Needling analgesia

It has been clear ever since the earliest days of neurophysiological research into needling that the response to needling is complex and that other transmitters are involved as well as opioids.

Serotonin is one transmitter that is important in the pain control matrix. Serotonin is involved in the brainstem in the activation of the descending pain inhibitory systems, and leads to the release of more serotonin (as well as nor adrenaline) in the dorsal horn, as discussed below (Han & Terenius 1982).

Stimulation of Aδ-nerve fibers may also activate the serotonergic and noradrenergic descending inhibitory system. Shah et al. found that the concentration of 5-HT and noradrenaline, was higher in the vicinity of active MTrPs compared to latent MTrP or normal muscle tissue. 5-HT receptors are primarily pronociceptive in the periphery, acting directly on afferent nerves and indirectly by release of other mediators (e.g., SP and glutamate).

Oxytocin may have an important role in many of the effects of dry needling, including analgesic, anxiolytic and sedative effects (Uvnas-Moberg et al 1993). Oxytocin release is also generated by stroking, gentle massage and physical touch, particularly to the ventral surface of the body.

Analgesia can be produced by shock in some animals. The shock may include painful electrical stimulation in experiments that are supposed to be investigating (non-painful) dry needling. The mechanism for this effect may be release of ACTH and β-endorphin from the pituitary into the circulation. This can lead to some confusion in interpreting the findings of laboratory studies of electro dry needling.

IV.   Descending inhibitory pain control

In contrast to segmental analgesia, needling also induces a generalized analgesia throughout the body. It does this by activating an area in midbrain from which bundles of fibers descend to every level of the spinal cord and inhibit the dorsal horn. The various pathways of descending inhibitory control can be seen in a composite drawing of the neurophysiology of dry needling.

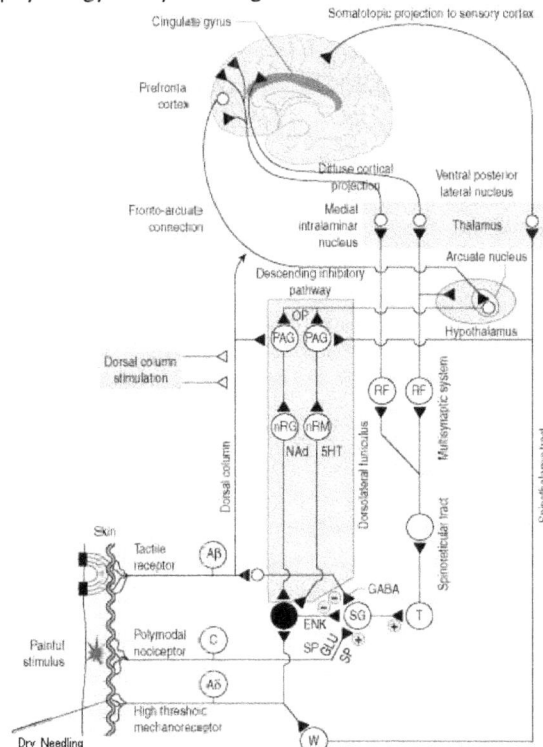

Figure 1: The afferent pathways involved in transmitting nociceptive information from a painful scar to the higher centers via the dorsal horn, the ascending tracts and the thalamus

The crucial structure for this descending pain inhibition is the periaqueductal grey (PAG), a small group of cells in the midbrain, and the nearest thing the body has to a 'pain control centre'. The PAG is the site at which the smallest dose of administered opioid drugs (e.g. morphine or heroin) can produce the most profound analgesic effect.

The PAG is activated by β-endorphin, which is released from nerve fibres descending from the hypothalamus, or more precisely the arcuate nucleus of the hypothalamus. The arcuate nucleus is also where some of the afferent pathways of the Aδ fibres, stimulated by dry needling, terminate. (The use of term 'Aδ' includes both the true Aδ fibres in skin and the type II/III fibres in muscle, which dry needling needles stimulate.) The PAG also receives input from the limbic system, which explains how psychological states can alter the perception of pain.

There are two known descending pathways from the PAG, and probably more that are yet to be discovered:

- One system descending from the PAG releases serotonin at the intermediate cells of the dorsal horn – the same cells that are already activated by the segmental effect of dry needling. The descending pain control system releases serotonin, stimulating the intermediate cell to release met-enkephalin, which in turn inhibits the substantial gelatinosa cells. This effect will be in addition to any segmental inhibition that is already active.
- Another descending pathway causes the release of noradrenaline diffusely throughout the dorsal horn. Noradrenaline has a direct inhibitory effect on the post-synaptic membrane of the transmission cells, further reinforcing the effect of dry needling on controlling nociception.

Descending inhibitory pain control inhibits the nociceptive pathway in every dorsal horn. These particular actions of needling might be influenced by pharmacological intervention. For example, tricyclic antidepressant drugs increase the release of both serotonin and noradrenaline in the central nervous system; there is some (admittedly not strong) evidence that tricyclic antidepressants may be synergistic with dry needling and increase its analgesic effect. Interestingly, this effect is not seen with the selective serotonin reuptake inhibitory drugs.

(2) Biochemical Modulation

(1) <u>Dry needling modulates the biochemicals associated with pain and inflammation (short term effects)</u>

The studies had shown that substance P, endorphin, and TNF were responsive to a short-term dry needling treatment. The effects on these biochemicals associated with pain and inflammation showed the following:

- Immediately after the 1 day treatment, an increase in the TNF levels in the muscle and the endorphin levels in the muscle and serum was accompanied by a reduction in the substance P levels of the muscle and DRG; and
- 5 days after the 1 day treatment, these variations in the substance P and endorphin levels were not observed, but TNF continued to accumulate along the needling path in the muscle through which the needle was manipulated in and out.

Shah et al. found the elevated levels of substance P in subjects with an active MTrP in the upper trapezius muscle during needle insertion. The elicitation of LTR resulted in a significant decrease in substance P concentration. The data obtained from different studies suggest that the dry needling treatment produces a short term analgesic effect by modulating the substance P and endorphin levels in peripheral sites.

A systematic review showed marked improvements in patients with MPS in which MTrPs were directly needled, suggesting that dry needling therapy has a specific efficacy in the treatment of pain arising from MTrPs. However, some clinical trials demonstrated that dry needling achieves only short term alleviation of pain and improvement of function. The biochemical changes may suggest that one mechanism by which short term dry needling produces brief analgesia in MPS may be the enhancement of peripheral endorphin in the serum and the muscle.

(2) <u>DN modulates the biochemicals associated with pain, inflammation and hypoxia (long-term effects)</u>

According to Yueh-Ling Hsieh et al, findings in addition to alterations of substance P, endorphin, and TNF; COX-2, HIF-1, iNOS, and VEGF were more responsive to long-term dry needing treatment. For these biochemicals associated with pain, inflammation, and hypoxia, the following was observed:

- Immediately after the 5 dose of treatment, TNF, iNOS, HIF-1, COX-2, VEGF, and substance P levels were enhanced in the needling-treated muscle, accompanied by an increase in substance P in the DRG and a reduction in serum endorphin level;
- After 5 days, these higher levels of TNF, iNOS, HIF-1, COX-2, VEGF, and substance P were maintained, whereas the endorphin levels in the muscle and serum increased. This result was supported by a study demonstrating that exercise induced muscle damage was associated with an increase in COX-2 and TNF levels.

TNF over expression was found in some traces of the needle penetrating into the muscle. Although TNF levels in the muscle and serum were enhanced by dry needling either in the 1 dose or the 5 dose treatment, abundant TNF accumulation and inflammatory cells were observed immediately and 5 day after the 5 dose treatment. The 5 dose treatment activated COX-2 level was also higher than the 1 dose treatment in the muscle. The increase in COX-2 expression was shown to be associated with the release of substance P, evoked by noxious stimuli from cultured DRG neurons. A more likely possibility is that 5 dose is an overloaded invasive manipulation to cause excess damage in the skeletal muscle fibers, stimulate excessive noxious inputs, and increase the release of substance P. The result of this study indicates that pain level was raised after long term dry needling. The results also showed that endorphin increases in 5 dose group 5 days after dry needling, but not immediately after dry needling. This result could be supported by a study demonstrating that the endorphin messenger RNA expression was more predominate in the later phases of inflammation (peaking on day 14), leading to attenuated pain responses. Whereas 5 doses increased the endorphin levels 5 days after ceasing treatment, the substance P levels in both the muscle and the DRG did not decrease. This result could be supported by a human study demonstrating that an increased level of endorphin is insufficient to inhibit pain in the temporomandibular joint.

(3) Mechanical effects

I. <u>Muscle damage</u>

Briefly, the usual sequence after muscle injury starts with the inflammatory reaction that removes cellular debris. Then, activated satellite cells, which become myoblasts, initiate a mitotic period. Next, the myoblasts fuse to create myotubes. In the cytoplasm of the myotubes, sarcomeres are synthesized. When the cytoplasm is filled with sarcomeres, the regeneration is complete.

Usually, minor damage to muscle triggers a rapid inflammatory response within the first 24 hours after injury, for example, physical exercise, crush plus heat, or chemical injury with bupivacaine. However, Allbrook described a mild mechanical injury which did not produce the inflammatory reaction until the fifth day. These authors lightly crushed the muscles with forceps applied for two minutes. The delay observed in the inflammatory reaction is because this was not a pure mechanical injury and vascular involvement also occurred.

Satellite cells typically reside on the surface of healthy adult muscle fibers. Satellite cells are undifferentiated "sleepers" stem cells waiting for the muscular lesions. When the muscle is attacked, satellite cells become myoblasts. As a result of the inflammatory reaction that follows after minimal lesion, the necrotized part of the sarcoplasm becomes a basal lamina cylinder. The first myoblast within this basal lamina cylinder is described usually about 24 hours after the injury, and then a period of mitoses of these stem satellite cells starts.

Myoblasts from satellite cells initiate a period of mitosis of 9 to 15 hours. The myoblasts resulting from this mitosis period fuse with each other and with the muscle fibers surrounding the area of injury. The resulting structure is a cell called a myotube.

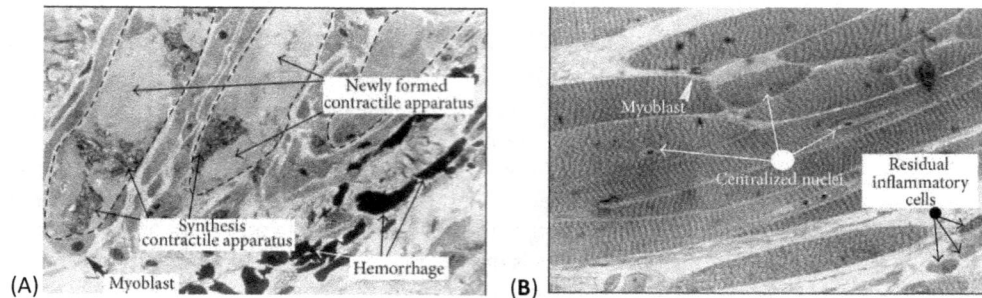

Figure 2: Muscle regeneration. (A) Myotubes. On the fifth day after puncture, (B) Young muscular fibers. Seven days after puncture. (Ares Domingo, , "Neuromuscular Damage and Repair after Dry Needling in Mice," Evidence-Based Complementary and Alternative Medicine, vol. 2013, Article ID 260806, 10 pages, 2013.)

Myotubes can be seen three days after eccentric running exercise in rats or four days after damage induced by lengthening contractions. In the stage of myotubes, actin and myosin are synthesized to create sarcomeres. The synthesis of actin and myosin is called myofibrillogenesis. The cytoplasm begins to be filled with sarcomeres about four days after exposure to bupivacaine or six days after crush injury. In much more aggressive injuries, such as a complete lesion of the whole muscle, sarcomeres may be observed by day seven. The myofibrillogenesis found in the post-DN treatment is similar in time periods to those obtained with other methods of injury.

When myofibrillogenesis is almost finished, the morphology of the regenerated area is like the normal muscle fiber: whole cytoplasmic volume occupied by sarcomeres and nuclei extruded to the periphery. However, some centralized nuclei can be observed in the regenerated area. This is a common finding after any muscle injury, also after DN.

In summary, the repetitive mechanical injury in the muscle fiber resembles the classical pattern previously described by other investigators in muscular regeneration. In addition, a skeletal muscle is a dynamic tissue with an extraordinary capacity for repair after an injury. TNF, iNOS, and VEGF are essential molecules involved in cellular events to activate the formation of new blood vessels and to repair the injured muscles. In a study, the 5 dose treatment enhanced the expression of these proteins, and thus, a 5 dose -induced muscle injury that can promote the rearrangement and repair of skeletal muscles with a taut band is of particular interest. Prevention of muscle fibrosis is the main objective of improving muscle healing following an injury from 5 dose treatment.

II. Nerve Injury

As common with muscle, the researchers have obtained images of nerve injury with DN. These nerve injuries follow the classic pattern of Wallerian degeneration, initial fragmentation nerve segments, followed by axonal phagocytosis. This phagocytosis at the synaptic level becomes synaptic contact abandoning which produces dispersion of the postsynaptic acetylcholine receptors.

The cascade of events that lead to axonal fragmentation occurs as follows (Stirling and Stys, 2010):

- Nerve section keeps the distal end without inputs of axoplasmic flow of substances and without axoplasmic transport of organelles;
- At 24 hours after injury, the distal axonal section already suffers from an energy deprivation; because of a lack of ATP, the ionic pumps (Na^+/K^+, Ca^{2+}) stop working with a net result of an influx of calcium; finally this calcium activates the calpain protease which degrades the axonal neurofilaments, and then fragmented axons can be seen.

During the first 24 hours after puncture, Schwann cells surround the axon segments to be digested; this phenomenon was described by Miledi and Slater. During this process, Schwann cells occupy the synaptic cleft contributing to the nerve terminal degeneration resulting in the glial phagocytosis is a synaptic contact abandoned by the axon.

As described by Thesleff, the synaptic component abandoned by degenerated axons cannot maintain aggregation of its postsynaptic receptors. These receptors tend to disperse on the myocyte surface. This situation, called "post denervation hypersensitivity," consists of an area larger than the synaptic contact and which is sensitive to acetylcholine molecules.

Finally, the proximal end of the injured axon elongates following the path of the remaining glia to reoccupy its postsynaptic component. The chemical stimulus favors axoplasmic flow and transport, and a distal dilatation that is responsible for axonal growth, called growth cone, appears. When the axons are broken within the muscle by injuries such as exercise, the nerve-muscle contact is quickly reestablished. The nerve injury with DN is made within the muscle, and the endplates newly reinnervated at the third day after puncture.

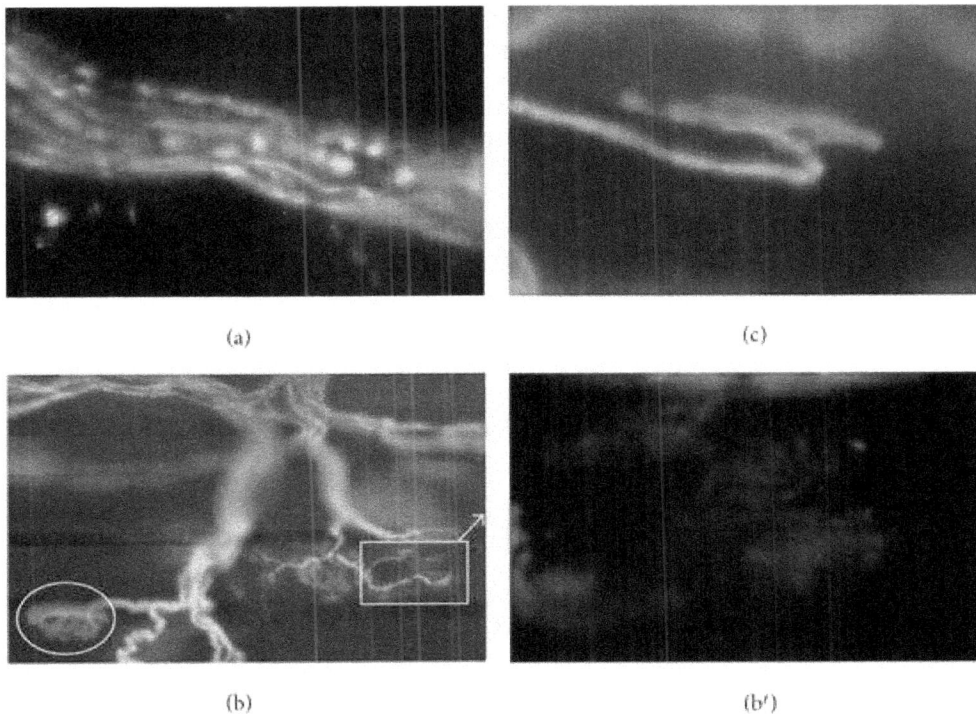

(a)

(c)

(b)

(b')

Figure 3: (a) Intramuscular nerve shows some axons with fragmented neurofilament, (b) The circle shows an example of normal endplate, (b'), this unstructured component, (c) Several days after completion of reinnervation, axonal regrowth, (Ares Domingo, , "Neuromuscular Damage and Repair after Dry Needling in Mice," Evidence-Based Complementary and Alternative Medicine, vol. 2013, Article ID 260806, 10 pages, 2013.)

A growth cone beyond its endplate is a common finding after reinnervation and becomes a residual for several days. The axonal growth cone can be seen at day three after puncture.

Axotomy is a complete nerve section which usually occurs with nerve endings separation (Bishop, 1982). However, DN induces only a partial lesion of the nerve branch without separation of the ends. The sites of experimental nerve injury are usually extramuscular (Verhaagen et al, 1988, and Lichtman, 1989), which makes both denervation and reinnervation slow. The nerve damaged by the repetitive mechanical injury is close to the neuromuscular synapse, and its fast reinnervation follows the classic patterns.

III.   Improves local blood flow and promotes healing

There is often some redness of the skin around the needled area during or after treatment, particularly on the trunk; a sign of the release of vasoactive neuropeptides including CGRP and histamine. Sometimes fluid extravasation also occurs and a weal can be seen, which is similar to that seen as a result of the release of histamine. The patient may feel itchiness.

Experiments have shown that the blood flow in the skin and muscle of healthy volunteers increases as soon as a needle is inserted into the skin, and increases further when the needle is advanced into the underlying muscle, and increases still further when the needle is stimulated and LTR is elicited (Sandberg et al 2003).

The local release of neuropeptides by dry needling can influence other structures in the vicinity. For example, dry needling on the face can affect the activity of salivary glands. Patients with dry mouth due to post-irradiation xerostomia recorded an increase in saliva production after dry needling the TrP around the salivary glands (Blom et al 1993).

More studies showed that HIF-1 up regulation can be induced not only by hypoxic stress but also mechanical stress. Induction of HIF target genes, including VEGF and iNOS, can promote angiogenesis, vasodilation, and altered glucose metabolism in hypoxic tissues. Studies using enhanced HIF-1 expression suggest that HIF-1 up regulation is a beneficial therapeutic modality for hypoxia/ischemia. The region containing numerous MTrPs can become focally ischemic because of limited oxygen supply by compression of the muscle contracture. Human studies also suggest that local, temporary hypoxia and blood flow reduction within muscle fibers in patients with trapezius myalgia, as well as the degree of hypoxia and impaired circulation, are correlated of pain intensity. Studies showed that the fry needling treatment can enhance HIF-1, iNOS, and VEGF production in the treated muscle. Thus, the increases in HIF-1protein levels can up regulate VEGF protein expression, potentially increasing capillarity in the skeletal muscle. Therefore, the expression of HIF-1, iNOS, and VEGF proteins can be key to improving circulation in muscles containing MTrPs after dry needling.

Understanding needle

Dry needle has five different parts i.e. tip, body, root, handle & tail.

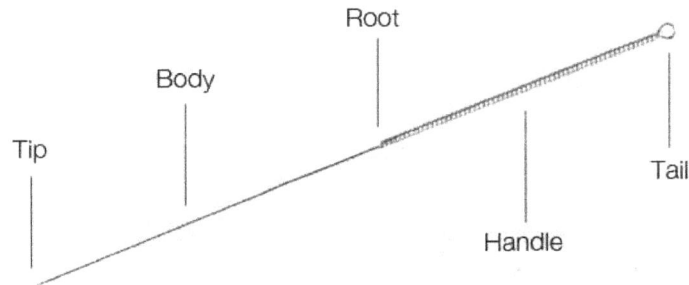

Figure 4: Anatomy of a needle

1. Needle tip: The part of the needle that is inserted into the skin. Researchers have shown that certain tip angle and types of edges can lessen the insertion force and can separate tissue differently.

2. Needle body: It is also called as shaft. It is made from surgical stainless steel wire of different thickness. Needles are so thin that they can be bent when touched at the needle tip. There are two ranges of needle available in the market, lower end and higher end. Higher end needle have low nickel content which is suitable for the patient with metal allergies.

3. Root: it is typically the part of the needle where handle and needle shaft unite. It is the weakest part of the needle.

4. Needle handle: therapist holds the handle to manipulate the needle in try to elicit LTR. They come in variety of color and are designed to ease the therapist in manipulation and grip. They may be pipe handled which is crimped at two or three locations to secure the handle to the shaft. They may be plastic molded handles which are color coded for easy identification of needle size and gauge or they may be wire wounded which is commonly used. Handle is created by winding the metal wire around the shaft. They may be looped or none looped at the tail.

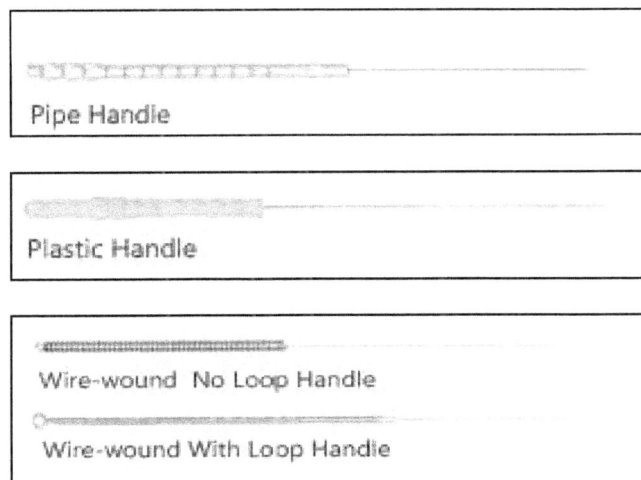

Figure 5: Type of needle handles.

5. Needle tail: therapist taps the needle through the guide tube at the tail only. It is flatten at the top or may be looped.

6. Guide tubes – guide tube as the name suggests guides the therapist in needle insertion. Guide tube encloses the needle and is open from both the sides, one end allowing the needle insertion into the skin while other end assisting the therapist taping the needle. Tube will retain the needle and preventing the needle from contamination. They vary in length and diameter depending upon the size of handle and length of the needle. They allow easy and quick insertion of the needle.

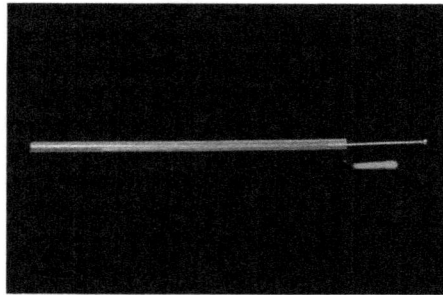

Figure 6: Guide tube

Handling the Needles

- Unwrapping the packet – needles must be unpacked immediately before the treatment begins. Sterile needles come in a individually sealed packing with normally 100 needles per box. To unwrap the needles therapist must hold the needle packet from the bottom and slowly peel the paper backing from top to bottom direction. Therapist must hold the needle from the handle along with guide tube, and any attempt to touch the needle body or tip should be avoided. Therapist must immediately move the needles into the sterile surface, or therapist may open one needle at a time required during the treatment process. If any needle during this process comes in contact with unsterile object, it must be discarded. If there is any open needle that is left unused after the treatment it must also be discarded.

- The needle should be handled with the shaft and the tip and the body of the needled should not be touched.

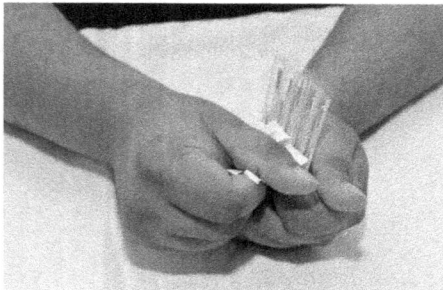

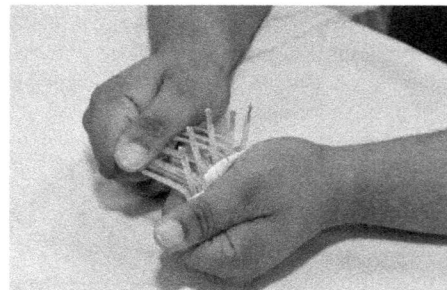

Figure 7: Unwrapping the needles

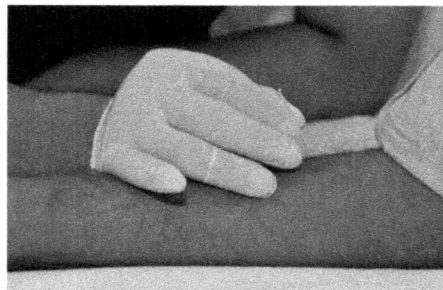

Figure 8: Holding the needle from shaft

Method of needling

Practicing needling

The correct knowledge of anatomy, palpation skills, clinical reasoning to diagnose condition structurally and application of correct techniques are some fundamental factors to achieve the desired results. Dry Needling procedure requires skillful trained hands, and the knowledge of correct techniques which can only be obtained with practice. Practicing allows the therapist to acquaint oneself with the needle, and to gain the confidence so that needling can be done in clinical practice very accurately, perfectly and with least complications. Certain complications which can be encountered with poor needling technique or inexperienced hands are bent needles, broken needles etc. During the practice session aim of the therapist is to learn proper needle insertion, manipulation techniques (like pistoning and rotating) along with needle withdrawal technique. After practicing therapist must be able to use the needle as painlessly as possible and manipulate it as per requirement. Practicing with the thin needles can be done in three steps:

1. Paper cushion and cotton pack practice:
    A. Paper cushion practice: To make a paper cushion, soft recycled papers are folded up to 30 to 50 layers to make a bundle of dimensions approx 2 to 3 cm thick, 5 to 8 cm wide, 5 to 8 cm long. The paper bundle is now fastened with a thread in form of double cross. This method is used to gain finger strength and to learn proper needle insertion and needle withdrawal technique. To practice this, therapist one hand holds the paper cushion while the other hand holds the needle keeping the body of the needle straight. As the needle touches the cushion, therapist's thumb and index finger rotates the needle forward and backward into the cushion alternatively and at the same time gently

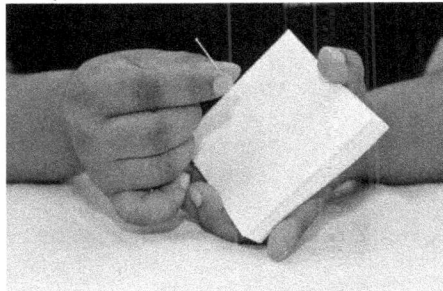

Figure 9: Paper cushion technique

pushing the needle into the paper cushion. Once inserted, to withdraw the needle from the punctured cushion, therapist must rotate the needle gently pulling the needle away from the paper cushion. After removal, this method is again repeated on other place away from the punctured site. This practice is pursued until the needle can be advanced into the cushion without bending and twirling, or till the needle insertion and withdrawal can be controlled freely. A needle can be manipulated 150 times/ min. During practice, the needle of smaller size (i.e. .25 X 25mm) should be used at first slowly progressing to longer sizes once the therapist has gained enough confidence and finger strength. To meet the clinical expertise therapist must continue to practice needling technique and with both the hands. This technique is used to practice needle insertion and withdrawal technique.

    B. Cotton pack: To make cotton pack for practice, the cotton roll is fastened by a thread into a ball of 6 to 8 cm in diameter. The pack is then wrapped by a piece of cloth. As the cotton pack is soft inside it can be used to practice manipulating the needle like lifting, rotating, inserting and withdrawing the needle. The therapist holds the needle with thumb and index finger and inserts the needle into the cotton ball slowly and gently to practice manipulating techniques. Insertion and withdrawal of the needle should be combined with rotation of the needle. This method enables the therapist to practice needling with proper depth and constant speed and to

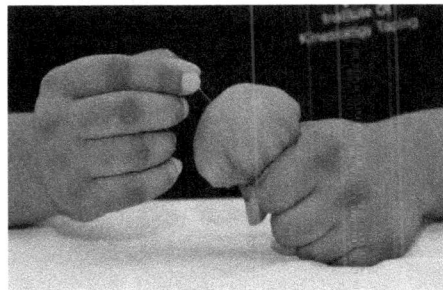

Figure 10: Cotton pack technique

rotate the needle with the same force and the same speed.

2. Practice on oneself :
After practicing on paper/cotton pack, therapist may practice the needling insertion and

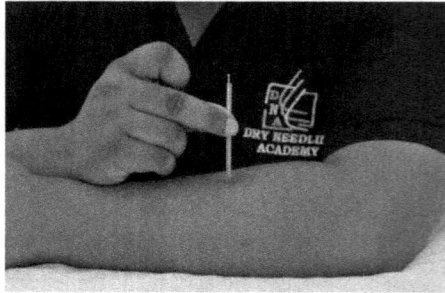

Figure 11: Practice on oneself technique

withdrawal techniques on oneself to experience the feeling of pin prick and response of the body during manipulation of the needle. While inserting, the body of the needle should be vertically straight, allowing smooth insertion while firmly gripping the needle. The manipulation should be flexible and even, also, the manipulation speed should be free. The therapist must establish a relationship between the finger strength and needle insertion, and between needle manipulation and feeling of the needled region.

3. Practice on others:
After practicing needling on oneself, it should be practiced on others like your colleagues to

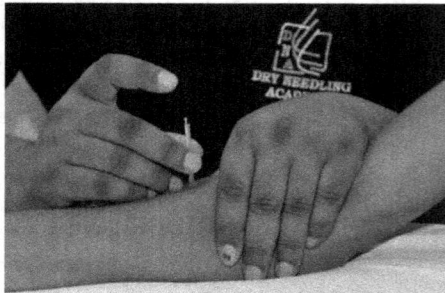

Figure 12: Practice on others technique

stimulate clinic practice. Since each individual is different, they may respond differently to the needling technique performed. This enables the therapist to observe wide range of results and responses of dry needling. Therapist must keep in mind not to bend the needle in order to insert it into targeted tissue or to change the direction of the needle. Instead therapist should withdraw the needle outside the tissue and reinsert it. Needle should always follow the simplest way inside the tissues to reach its target. Aim to practice needling should be it should be harmonious, skillful and freely.

Direction/angle of insertion

Needling requires skillful insertion of the needle in the correct direction to get the desired effect i.e. tonification and sedation. Not only direction but depth of insertion and angle of insertion is also important which depends on factors like anatomical site, etc. Ideally needle can be inserted between 15 degrees to 90 degrees. Angle of the needling depends on the structures underlying the targeted area. There are three main techniques used by the therapist:

- Perpendicular insertion: needle is inserted almost perpendicular to the skin. Most of the trigger points are treated with this technique only. This is useful where the underlying tissue is thick i.e. muscle.
- Oblique insertion: used to treat thin muscles and to avoid the underlying structures. The needle is inserted at an approx angle of 45 degrees to the skin. As in case of upper trapezius needling, the therapist must use an oblique insertion technique to avoid injury to lobe of lung hence preventing pnemothorax.
- Third technique is inserting the needle almost parallel to the skin; forming an angle of 10 to 15 degrees to the skin. This is commonly used while treating the very thin muscle like muscle of head or the thorax to avoid cardiac tamonade, or pnemothorax.

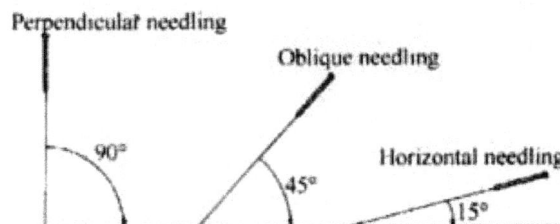

Figure 13: Insertion angles

Basic insertion techniques

Therapist uses both his hand to insert the needle, one hand may hold the guide tube (assisting hand) on the tissue while other hand simply taps the needle through the guide tube (needling hand). Other techniques may insist the therapist to use one hand to press the skin, to hold up the tissue or to stretch the skin while the other hand holds the guide tube as well as tap the needle simultaneously with appropriate speed, depth and direction. He then removes the guide tube and follows the further treatment.

1. Finger Press Insertion:
   Gently presses beside the trigger point with the nail of the thumb and index finger of assisting hand while the other hand holds the needle. Now keep the needle tip closely against the finger nail of assisting hand, and insert the needle into the trigger point. This method is appropriate for short needles.

2. Pinched Needle Insertion:
   Wrap the needle body with a sterilized cotton ball by the thumb and the index finger of assisting hand, leaving 0.2-0.3 cm of its tip exposed, and hold the needle handle with the thumb and index finger of the other hand. As the needle tip is directly over the trigger point, insert the needle swiftly into the skin with both hands. This method is appropriate for long needles.

3. Stretched Skin Insertion:
   Stretch the skin where the trigger point is located with the thumb and index finger of one hand, hold the needle with the other hand and insert it into the point rapidly to a certain depth. This method is appropriate for the points on the abdomen where the skin is loose.

4. Pinched Skin Insertion:
   Pinch the skin up around the trigger point with the thumb and index finger of assisting hand; insert the needle rapidly into the trigger point with the needling hand into the pad formed by pinching. This method is appropriate for puncturing the points on the face, where the muscle and skin are thin.

The needle insertion sensation varies greatly from person to person. It may vary from simple pin pinprick to tingling sensation or a muscle cramp. A healthy muscle will have a little discomfort during the insertion of the needle but a shortened muscle or a muscle will active trigger point may produce symptoms or referred pain upon insertion. It is a diagnostic as well as therapeutic indicator for the treating therapist that he hit the spot **RIGTH!** Whereas it is important for the patient to welcome and get used to those unpleasant felling felt during needling to deactivate the trigger point.

Manipulation of the needle

The aim of the dry needling is to elicit local twitch response (LTR) to deactivate active trigger points, to reduce pain, to regain original muscle length and function. After needle insertion, needle is manipulated in up and down motion (pistoning technique) ;or is moved in clockwise or anticlockwise direction (rotation technique) in pursuit to elicit LTR. This procedure may take a brief to several minutes depending on the clinical situations.

LTR constitute abrupt contraction of the muscle followed by relaxation. Generating brisk and vigorous pathognomic twitches relieves pain. In acute situations, there is hyper-excitability of the MTrPs and the twitches are strong enough to lift the joint upon which the stimulated muscle acts, in an anti-gravity fashion, and the twitches can even fatigue abruptly. In chronic situations, MTrPs are very difficult to find and the twitches tend to be of low force. Acute problems without underlying chronic problems have excellent prognosis and chronic problems tend to have guarded prognosis from presence of partial nerve and muscle fibrosis.

During manipulation there is twisting and aggregation of collagen fibers around the needle. This twisting and aggregation of collagen fibers activates a cellular response in fibroblasts which lasts up to several centimeters away from manipulation site. This transduction of mechanical signals into fibroblasts leads to a variety of extracellular and cellular events, neuromodulation and healing. Also increased cortisol levels in the tissue stimulate scar tissue breakdown and tissue remodeling.

Order of insertion and removal of needles

It is always beneficial to plan the treatment beforehand. It is important to count the number of needles to be inserted. One can note them in their notes the number of needles used to avoid complication of forgotten needles. Please ensure that all the needles are removed. Needle can be inserted / removed in following order:

- Above downward;
- Proximal to distal;
- Away from or towards the therapist;
- Less painful to more painful points.

Retaining needles

The needles can be retained in the position from 10 minutes to a maximum of 30 minutes. If the patient cannot tolerate retention, the needles can be stimulated immediately and can be withdrawn immediately.

Removal of needles

Removal of the needles should be rapid. A piece of cotton should be kept in assisting hand while dominant hand removes the needles in order to provide compression in case of any bleeding and to avoid contact with blood if bleeding occurs.

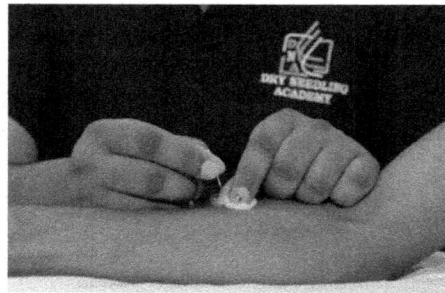

Figure 14: Removal of needle

The Procedure

Patients Education

Before starting the treatment it is important for the therapist to inform the patient about different aspects of dry needling. Proper education of the patient is necessary as it helps the therapist to gain patient's confidence, to achieve relaxation of the body part to be treated, to get appropriate feedback from the patient throughout the treatment process. Patient must be enlightened about:

1. Difference between dry needling and acupuncture.
2. Patient must be informed about aims, nature and indications of treatment.
3. Patient must be familiarized about the techniques and needles used in the treatment.
4. He must be taught about the expected reactions during the treatment like pinprick, dull pain or reproduction of his symptoms.
5. He must be told about some unwanted signals that are common during the treatment like numbness, strong pain, burning sensation.
6. He must be taught about the importance of his response during the entire treatment and the need to keep his body relaxed during the treatment.
7. Patient must be informed that he may stop the treatment at any time if he wants by using verbal cues.
8. Any questions from the patient are welcomed, and therapist must ensure that the patient is well satisfied and has no further queries.
9. He must also be told about some adverse effects of dry needling like drowsiness, muscle soreness, or small haematomas.

Hygiene

Since dry needling is an invasive procedure, maintaining the hygiene throughout the procedure is utmost important. Even a small negligence may lead to infection at the puncture site. All the major infections including HIV, Hepatitis B, may result from errors in maintenance of hygiene. Only trained professional is allowed to conduct the procedure under strict guideline as provided by their Nation. These best practices are measures that have been determined through scientific evidence or expert consensus most effectively to protect patients, health care providers, and communities.

Hygiene and infection control guidelines are mentioned below to be taken care of while performing the procedure.

1. General Infrastructure Requirements:
   Dry Needling procedure must be clean and be capable of being kept clean. A smooth impervious floor is preferable to a carpeted one, though the latter is acceptable. A hot and cold wash basin fitted with foot- or elbow-operated taps is essential. The basin should be cleaned with a suitable household non-abrasive cream at the end of each session. Soap and disposable paper towels must be available and accessible; hot air hand dryers are also acceptable. Lighting must be adequate. Other operating surfaces should likewise have a smooth impervious surface and must be kept clean.
2. Couch:
   The surface of the couch should have a smooth impervious surface, such as vinyl, in good repair. It should be kept clean and washed with detergent and hot water regularly. Patients should lie on a disposable paper sheet rather than the bare surface. Sheet must be replaced after every treatment session.
3. Therapist's Hygiene:
   Good personal hygiene is important. Hands must be clean with nails short and clean. He must avoid using artificial nails or extender during the treatment. If the therapist has a cut or abrasion, or any type of skin infection, on his wrist or hand, he must use gloves. It is not necessary to use sterilized surgical gloves: vinyl examination gloves are cheaper, and serve the purpose. A new pair should be used after each client. Broken skin or infections on other exposed parts of body, such as face, should be covered with a waterproof bandage.
   A. Therapist's hand hygiene:
      Hand hygiene and skin integrity of therapist: Perform hand hygiene (i.e. wash or disinfect hands) before preparing needling material and treatment. The need for hand hygiene

between each session will vary depending on the setting and whether there was contact with soil, blood, or body fluids.

a. Indications for hand washing:

- Therapist must wash hands if they are visibly dirty, or contaminated with blood or other body fluids. He must decontaminate his hands if it comes in direct contact with patient's non intact skin.
- Therapist must decontaminate his hands before any direct contact with the patient, and before starting the needling procedure.
- Therapist must wash his hands before and after the treatment and before wearing and after removing gloves.
- Therapist must decontaminate his hands after touching any object (including medical equipment) in immediate vicinity of the patient during the treatment procedure.
- Decontamination of hands is must if moving from a contaminated body site to clean body site of the patient during the treatment procedure.
- Therapist must decontaminate his hands before and after using the restroom.

b. Types of Hand wash:
- Therapist must wash his hand with antimicrobial soap and water or with a non antimicrobial soap and water, before and after the treatment as they limit the bacterial growth.
- Alternatively therapist may use alcohol based hand rubs routinely to decontaminate his hands in clinical setting if hands are not visibly soiled.
- Washing hands with non antimicrobial soap and water is considered as an alternative to using antimicrobial impregnated wipes as it is not considered efficient enough to reduce bacterial counts as compared to alcohol based hand rubs or antimicrobial soap and water.

Good   **Better**   **Best**

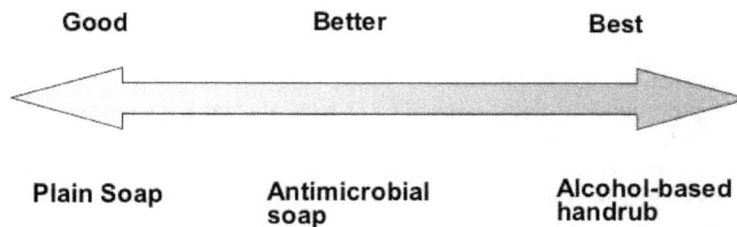

Plain Soap   **Antimicrobial**   **Alcohol-based**
                  soap   **handrub**

Figure 15: type of hand hygiene product with their importance.

c. Hand Hygiene Technique:

- Always follow the manufacturer's recommendations regarding the volume of the product to be used.
- If using alcohol based hand rubs, apply the product to the palm and then rub hands together covering all dorsal and palmer surfaces of both the hand and fingers until hands are dry.
- If using soap and water to decontaminate hands always wet the hands first followed by application of the product as per manufacturer recommendation and rub for at least 15 minutes covering all the surfaces of both the hands and fingers. Then rinse the hand and dry thoroughly with a disposable towel.
- Therapist must avoid using hot water repeatedly as it may increase the risk of dermatitis.

- Use of disposable towel is recommended. Use of liquid soaps or leaflet is acceptable but if using bar soap then it recommended to use smaller bars.
- After washing hands therapist must use a moisturizer if his hands are dry to minimize the incidence of irritant contact dermatitis related with repeated hand washing or hand antisepsis.

4. Equipments Hygiene:
- Only use sterile single use individually packed needles. Use a sterile needle for each treatment Inspect packaging for breaches in barrier integrity. Discard a needle or syringe if the package has been punctured, torn, or damaged.
- Bin to dispose of Paper tissues/cotton.
- "Sharps" disposable boxes for used or contaminated needles;
- Sterilized metal forceps to manage adverse events like stuck needle etc;
- Pre-packed alcohol-impregnated swabs,
- Disinfectants to decontaminate hands in between the treatment
- Always use a sterile pair of glove for each patient.

5. Hygiene During Preparation:
   a) Skin preparation: The patient's clothes should remain well away from the area of the skin to be pierced. An alcohol impregnated swab should be used to disinfect the skin before needling commences. If swabbing is done with an antiseptic use a clean, single-use swab and maintain product-specific recommended contact time. Do not use cotton balls stored wet in a multi-use container. Visibly soiled or dirty skin should be washed. Needling should not be carried out within 6 inches of infected areas of skin or body, or areas covered with skin rash. It should be deferred until the infection has cleared or the rash has been treated adequately.
   b) Preparation of material:
      1. Needles must not be kept on any non-sterile surface prior to use but they must be directly used from the sterile pack.
      2. If any unused needle comes in contact with the skin, nail, or any non-sterile surface it must be discarded immediately in disposable container without using it for the treatment.
      3. If the sterile needle pack is torn or used needle must be discarded.
   c) After care:
      - Disposable needles: These must be placed immediately after each patient's treatment is completed in a suitable sharps disposable box. Forceps should also be re-autoclaved after every session.
      - Paper towels and swabs: Must be renewed between patients. Used towels and swabs must be placed in a lidded plastic-lined bin.
      - Care of skin after needling: The punctured area of skin should be left uncovered.

6. Hygienic procedure for needling
   The following list of step-by-step procedures, based on the directions given above, may be helpful.
   A. Before each session
      i. Estimate number of needles to be used for the next day or session.
      ii. Set out the disposable needles, without removing them from their packets,
      iii. Autoclave forceps and container.
      iv. Clean down table and/or couch surfaces as instructed.
   B. Before commencing needling
      v. Wash and dry hands.
      vi. Place large fresh paper towel on table surface and/or couch.
      vii. Clean skin with spirit swab.

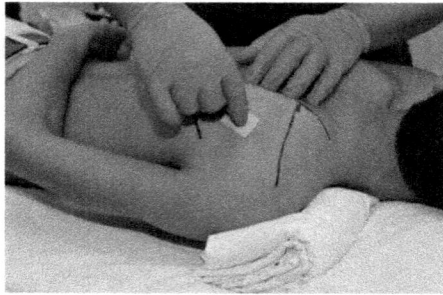

Figure 16: Cleaning the treatment field/ area.

C. After needling

viii. When needling is finished, remove needle from patients, place disposable needles in "sharps" disposal box.

ix. Do not cover puncture spots.

x. Remove disposable paper/ bed sheet and all swabs or tissues used on patient, place it in bin.

xi. Clean down table surfaces.

xii. Wash and dry hands.

7. Disposal

All waste matter (except needles) like swabs, paper towels and tissue should be collected in a sealable leak-proof plastic bag or box and incinerated, or autoclaved before disposal. Particular care must be taken in the disposal of needles; a stout, sharps disposal box for needles, such as is used in hospitals, is recommended; enclosed sharps container that is puncture-proof and leak-proof and that is sealed before it is completely full. Seal sharps containers for transport to a secure area in preparation for disposal. After closing and sealing sharps containers, do not open, empty, and reuse them. Manage sharps waste in an efficient, safe, and environment-friendly way to protect people from voluntary and accidental exposure to used equipment. Prevent access to the used needles. Disinfectants may be poured carefully down the sink after use, and flushed with running water. All other items used for one customer e.g. paper tissues, paper cups etc., must be disposed of into a waste bin lined with a plastic bag which can be sealed and incinerated. Special arrangements must be made for disposal of the sharps boxes and sealed waste-bags which should not be allowed to enter the public refuse collection system. Most Environmental Health Departments will be pleased to offer advice and possibly, assistance.

Materials required

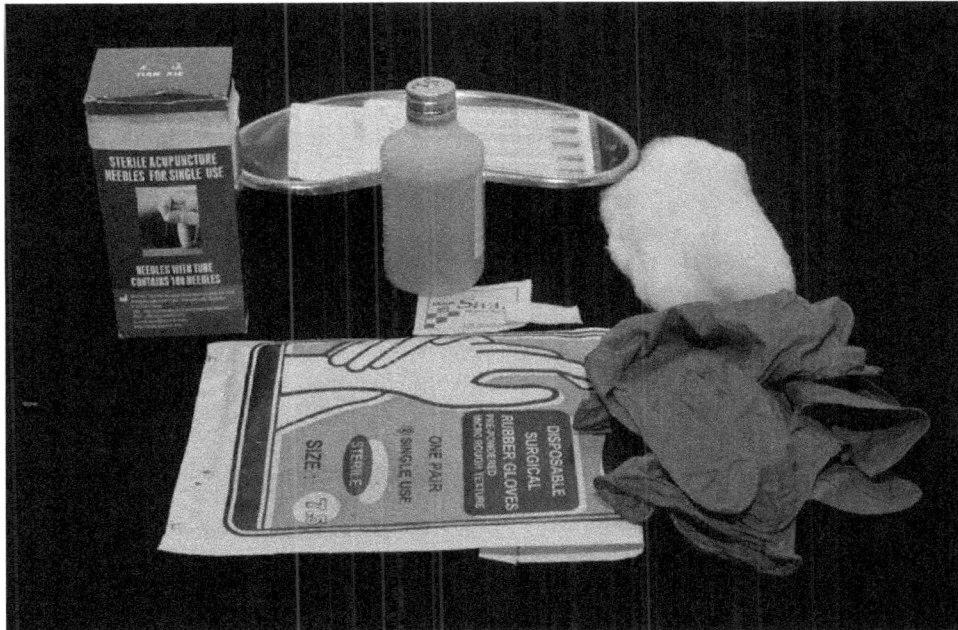

Figure 17: Materia required for dry needling procedure

- Needles: Dry needling is performed with sterile needles. Needles are available in different types, lengths, and diameters. The needles are made of stainless steel and have a relatively low nickel content to minimize possible allergic reactions.
- Disinfectants: Although the risk of infection is minimal with dry needling, we do recommend disinfecting the skin with either a cohol or isopropanol prior to needling.
- Needle Collectors Used needles are discarded in a needle collector. Regulations may vary in different countries. Practicing therapist must familiarize themselves with the regulations in their respective jurisdictions.
- Gloves Wearing (surgical) gloves is mostly to protect the clinician. In case of an accidental needle stick, a glove provides an additional barrier to anybody fluids and reduces the risk of infection. We recommend using a glove at least for the palpating hand.
- Swabs/Band-aids Occasionally there may be minor venous or arterial bleeding after removing the needle from the skin. Having swabs readily available helps in controlling the bleeding with compression. Compression is applied for approximately 1 minute, followed by a band-aid as needed.

Indication
- For the deactivation of active trigger points.
- For tonification of the muscle.
- To treat pain of muscular origin.
- To treat body structural impairment, pain and functional limitation.
- Restricted range of motion, contracture muscle fiber, and taut bands.
- To correct fascia adhesion or scar tissue.
- In conditions like: radiculopathies, joint dysfunction, disk pathology, tendonitis, migraines, tension-type headaches, carpal tunnel syndrome, spinal dysfunction, pelvic pain nocturnal cramps, etc.

Contraindications

Dry needling must be performed with caution. Therapist must choose the suitable patient for dry needling. The selection of patient should be done in relation to the patient's characteristics, medical history, clinical reasoning, likely benefits of the treatment, and whether the goals can be met with non-invasive treatments. In certain conditions dry needling is not permitted to be practiced.

- Needle phobia – if patient has needle phobia, then he is not a suitable patient for dry needling.
- Patient unwilling – if patient has some fear, or belief or reluctant to the treatment it should be avoided. For this therapist must inform patient all the benefits and risk of dry needling but must not try to persuade the patient to a dry needling treatment.
- Paresthesia- Patients with significant paresthesia must not be treated with dry needling as they are incapable of adequate feedback.
- Unable to give consent – if patient is unable to give consent due to communication, cognitive, age-related factors, avoid dry needling.
- Medical emergency or acute medical condition- All acute emergencies and life threatening emergencies must get medical treatment and must not be treated with dry needling.
- Acute infections/ Fever- Patients with acute systemic infections must not be treated with dry needling, as the reaction of dry needling treatment cannot be seen in advance and the patients should be in medical care.
- Compromised immune system - Increased risk of infections e. g. HIV.
- Blood thinning - Patients with vascular disease (e.g. hemophilia), or on blood thinning medications are more susceptible to hematoma and bleeding. Bleeding and bruising are among the most common side-effects of needling therapies. So these patient are not the candidate for dry needling.
- Lymph edema Lymph edema is also contraindication as the infection risk in the area of the lymph edema is increased immensely. For this reason it is suggested that there should be no dry needling in the affected area of the body following a surgical removal of a lymph node.
- Gravidity - 20–25% of pregnancies may naturally terminate in the first trimester and therefore erroneous connections between such occurrences and dry needling are possible. So pregnant patients must be treated with great caution. If a dry needling treatment is administered, the patient must give permission.
- Children- In addition to gaining informed consent from persons under 18 years old, parental or guardian consent in addition must be sought. Therapist must also ensure that the child is mature enough to understand the instruction given by the therapist.
- Psychiatric diseases - Some patients with psychological disorders or distress may not be optimal candidates for dry needling. High stress may reduce the likelihood of response to treatment and may increase risk of adverse psychological or physical response to dry needling. Also anxiety and emotional distress may impact on the ability to safely apply dry needling. Psychiatric patients are to be treated with dry needling only if the patient agrees and understands the procedure and risks of dry needling, can interpret the stimuli correctly and can give his full consent.
- Patient allergies – Patients allergic to metals may react to metals used in monofilament needles, particularly to nickel and chromium. A typical monofilament needle contains approximately 8–10% nickel and 11% chromium. So dry needling must be avoided.
- Epilepsy - In patients with epilepsy, caution should be taken due to intolerance of the patients to strong sensory stimulation. Patients with epilepsy should not be left unattended when needles are in situ and must be treated with care.
- Diabetes- Patients with diabetes may have compromised tissue healing capabilities, sensory deficits, and poor peripheral circulation. Diabetes may influence the decision to use needle or which needling techniques to use, e.g. superficial dry needling versus deep dry needling, and may determine the intensity of the treatment.
- Osteo synthesis and joint replacement Due to an increased risk of infection, dry needling should not be applied in the immediate vicinity of an osteo synthesis or a joint replacement due to reduced immune reaction. Any form of implant is an absolute contraindication. Needle contact with an implant must be avoided.
- Cardiac pacemaker Patients with a cardiac pacemaker must not be treated with dry needling.
- Contagious diseases Patients with infectious diseases (through blood) should be treated with special precaution.

- Severe pulmonary diseases Patients with a severe pulmonary disease should not be treated near the thorax.
- Mucous membranes, eyes, genitals – are the sensitive areas where dry needling should be avoided.

Precautions

- Only sterile single use needle should be used.
- Needle should not be expired or rusted or seal should not be broken.
- Treatment area should be sterile and clean.
- Treatment area should provide adequate privacy to the patient.
- Patient should be well aware of the procedure.
- Therapist must be well equipped to handle any adverse events, common during dry needling.
- Therapist must document the number of needle used, response of the patient during the process and progression in the treatment for every patient.
- Therapist must ensure that all needles are removed.
- He must not over needle the patient.
- To prevent the risk of a nerve injury therapist must make a run of the nerve. The needle must advance the muscle slowly and must be removed immediately if patient feels any shooting or burning pain. Therapist must pincer grip the muscle before needling.
- To prevent risk of injury of blood vessels-therapist must be well aware of the anatomical landmarks and the main arteries. He must localize the superficial vessel around the treatment area. Pincers grip the needled muscle if possible.
- Needling around joints: risk of intra-articular infection is high. It is important for the therapist to know the exact position of joint capsule. If possible needling around the joint is avoided or only superficial dry needling is used.
- Needling around thorax: only one side of the thorax should be needled at one session. A bilateral pneumothorax must be avoided. The danger zones of thorax are lungs. Special care must be taken to while needling round rib and facet joints. Therapist must use superficial dry needling technique, pincer grip the muscle, and tangentially approach the muscle.
- The abdominal muscles should be treated with dry needling only if; it is possible to grasp the muscle into a pincer grip to protect the internal organs. The rectus abdominis muscle is treated from lateral, tangentia to the abdomen. The quadratus lumborum muscle is consequently treated behind the retroperitoneum in the frontal plane. The needle tip should not be moved ventral towards the abdomen or cranial towards the lung.
- Palm and sole are the sensitive areas of hand and foot as nerves and blood vessels are too close to each other. Injury to this structure is common in hand and foot. Hence needling palm and sole must be avoided, and if needling thin needles is used.

Appropriate selection of patient

It is important for the therapist to choose the appropriate patient for the dry needling, not every patient is a suitable candidate for dry needling. This may come with experience and thorough knowledge.

1. Therapist must ensure therapeutic aim of patient and if dry needling corresponds to the desired outcome.
2. Consider the needs of dry needling or other factors like age/medical and psychological status of patient before needling.
3. Therapist must consider the medical condition of the patient this includes pregnancy, pacemaker, blood thinning medications.
4. Therapist must also consider patient ability to understand the process/nature of treatment and as well as the importance of the treatment.
5. Patient should be able to effectively communicate his responses during the treatment.
6. Patient should be able to comply with the requirement of treatment (lying still/no coughing/no laughing or be relaxed) and should be able to give consent for the treatment.

Procedure of Dry Needling

Before starting the treatment, therapist must goes through the checklist of indications and contraindications. After this he must ensure that patient is fully aware of the nature of treatment and has no queries regarding the treatment. Therapist must ensure that patient is willing for the procedure and can give a written consent form. Along with this therapist must ensure that the patient is a suitable candidate for dry needling. Dry needling procedure should always be followed step by step and in no hurry to avoid any complications. Before starting the treatment all the material required during the treatment should be collected at one sterile place and treatment room should be well equipped which includes fresh bed sheet, dustbin near the bed etc. The entire hygiene requirement must be fulfilled by the therapist. Therapist must plan the treatment in advance, and have an approximately idea of number and size of needles used and must have a thorough knowledge of underlying structures.

1. Patient Position - it is advisable to treat patient in lying position. He must be as relaxed as possible. He must be in a comfortable position with the support of pillows and cushions. Only treatment area should be exposed while other area should be draped with a cloth. Treatment room must provide patient adequate privacy. It is recommended for the therapist to see the face of the patient throughout the treatment to watch their reactions, but if this is not possible verbal communication will do.

2. Therapist's Position - Therapist must position himself is comfortable sitting position and close to the treatment area in order to hold the needle still, and to palpate the muscle precisely. All the material should be within one arm length reach and to the side of his dominant hand so that he can reach for anything without any difficult i.e. Needles, disposable container, alcohol swabs, gloves etc.

3. Palpation - therapist before starting the treatment must identify the anatomical landmarks. Then the muscle to be treated is identified. Now aim of the therapist should be to palpate any taut band, trigger points and an estimation of depth of trigger point and their numbers.

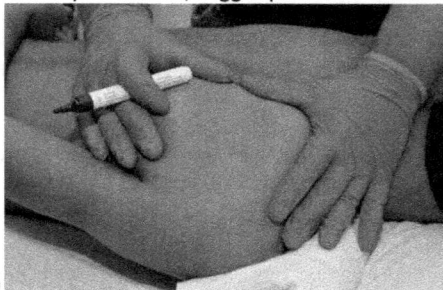 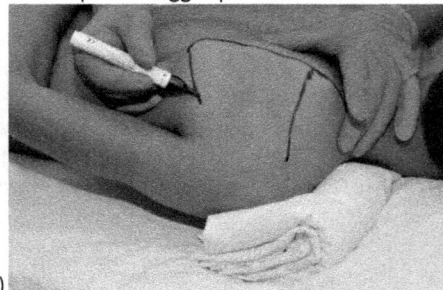

(A)   (B)

Figure 18:(A) Palpation of Anatomical landmarks , (B) Marking the Anatomical landmarks

4. Needling The Area -
   - After fulfilling all the hygiene requirements treatment should continue.
   - Therapist must clean the treatment area with disinfectant before every needle puncture. With the assisting hand therapist holds the muscle with pincer grip or flat palpation while the needling hand holds the needle from the shaft only. Any contact beyond the shaft is avoided.
   - Keeping all the vulnerable structures in mind therapist should advance the needle into the tissue slowly and easily. He must be prepared for sudden movement by the patient and for this reason therapist should stabilise his needling hand on the patient.
   - Therapist must use the needles size appropriately.
   - After the insertion of the needle into the taut band an attempt to elicit LTR is made. This is carried out with controlled manipulation of the needle. During this the needle must never leave the area between the landmarks, marked in advance.
   - Needle should advance the tissue at ease. Therapist must choose the direction and angle of needling to avoid injury to internal structures. If therapist faces any resistance in the tissue, he must withdraw and reinsert the needle again. Feedback from the patient is important throughout the procedure.

- When a LTR is elicited then the needle can be left in place till the cramp eases SDN or needle may be moved repeatedly up or down into the taut band until the cramp ceases or lessens DDN.
- If superficial Dry Needling is applied, the patient may be left by himself for a short period of time. The patient must be able to attract the attention of the therapist at all time.
- The patient must be capable of describing the various pains experienced throughout the treatment to the therapist. If this is not possible, it is not permitted to practice DN. If there is a burning or pricking pain after puncturing the skin, the direction of the needle must be altered in order to release the pain. After treatment the needle must be disposed of in the medical sharps collector. If bleeding starts after the removal of the needle, the area must be compressed with swabs until the bleeding stops.

5. Post Treatment – Stretching and cryotherapy of the muscle post needle is essential for an effective needle therapy. All the appropriate measures to ease the pain after a DN treatment should be explained to the patient.

Advantages
- It is minimally invasive therapy that relieves pain associated with muscles.
- It is quick to perform and is time efficient.
- It Improves joint mobility and reduces muscle tightness.
- In competent hands it is a safe treatment.
- It facilitates return of the patients to fully functional activities.
- It is equal to any than other manual techniques.
- Less treatment sessions required to aid recovery, hence cost effective.

Management of adverse events
Dry needling being an invasive procedure poses certain risks like bleeding, brusing, infection etc. These events or risks are termed as adverse events. A therapist must have knowledge of these adverse events and must be competent enough to deal with all of the adverse events efficiently. These adverse events may be described as mild, significant and serious all depending upon their severity.

- Pain during treatment
  If excessive pain persists while the needle is inserted it should be removed. If pain persists when the needle is inserted which is not consistent with the 'trigger point referred pain' (eg: sharp shooting pain or paresthesia) the needle should be removed. If pain persists following a treatment, the patient can be advised to apply heat or ice. If patient complains of pain while needling, therapist must give a quick check on the needle size, especially the length and gauge, and the insertion technique also.
- Injuries of nerves, veins and arteres
  Serious injuries as a result of dry needling are rare. However, superficial venous and arterial bleedings are fairly common. Generally, they are harmless, but may result in hematoma. Care should be taken to avoid injuring blood vessels, however if bleeding does occur, apply pressure to the area with a cotton swab after the needle has been withdrawn. Ice can be used locally to minimize the bruising. To prevent further bleeding the clinician should apply direct compression, especially in those patients taking anti-coagulants. Occasionally, clinicians may hit a nerve, which will result in sharp shooting pain down an extremity. Hitting a nerve normally does not cause any damage to the nerve. To minimize the risk of injury, the clinician must have an impeccable knowledge of anatomy. At all times, the therapist must know where and in what structure the tip of the needle moves.
- Fainting
  Dizziness and vertigo, sudden and excessive perspiration, or fainting may occur occasionally. This may be caused by nervous tension, hunger, fatigue, incorrect positioning, and excessive stimulation of the needles or if the patient is autonomically labile. To avoid fainting explain the procedure before treatment, treating the patient in a lying position may be preferable,

don't insert too many needles and use minimal stimulation on the first treatment. If fainting occurs stop needling and remove all needles, make sure the patient is lying down and consider raising their legs, offer water, warm tea or something sweet to eat and reassure the patient. Symptoms should abate after resting.

- Excessive drowsiness
  A small percentage of patients may feel excessively relaxed and sleepy after treatment. They should be advised not to drive until they have recovered. In such patients it is recommended that needle retention time is reduced and to apply milder stimulation.

- Stuck needle
  If the patient is not relaxed or apprehensive to the treatment this will result in a stuck needle. To avoid this it is mandatory for the therapist to explain the process to the patient, gain confidence of the patient and make him as much relax as possible. A stuck needle may occur due to spasm of the local muscle after insertion of the needle, twisting the needle with too much amplitude or in only one direction causing the muscle fibers to bind, or if the patient alters their position whilst the needles are in-situ. To avoid, position the patient in a relaxed manner, avoid excessive twisting of the needle and avoid needling tendinous muscle tissue. If the needle is stuck due to over rotation, then rotate the needle in the opposite direction and remove. If it is stuck due to muscle tension, leave the needle in for a short time, relax the tissue around the needle with massage, ice massage or by inserting 1-2 needles around the stuck needle, then remove the needle.

- Bent needle
  A needle may bend if it strikes hard tissue, if there is a sudden change in the patient's posture, or strong contraction of the muscle occurs during trigger point needling. To prevent this, insert the needle carefully with the patient in a comfortable position. If the needle does bend, instruct the patient not to move, relax the local muscle and remove the needle slowly following the course of the line of the bend.

- Broken needle
  This may occur due to poor quality of the needle, strong muscle spasm, sudden movements by the patient when the needle is in place or by withdrawing a bent needle. The most likely place for a needle to break is at the junction of the handle and the needle shaft. Clinicians should avoid inserting the needle all the way to the handle. The likelihood of a broken needle is very rare with the use of single use sterile needles as there is no metal fatigue from repeated use and autoclaving. The patient should be advised to remain calm to avoid the needle from going deeper. If the broken needle is exposed remove the broken section with tweezers, if it is not exposed press the tissue around the insertion site until the broken section is exposed and remove with tweezers. If the needle can't be remove in the clinic, medical attention must be sought so that the needle can be removed surgically.

- Infection
  The skin in the region to be needled should be inspected and if infection is suspected needling should be deferred and medical advice sought. Care should be taken when needling very thin or fragile skin. Infections can result in other serious complications such as erysipelas (a type of bacterial skin infection generally caused by group a streptococci) or viral infections. Extra caution is indicated in those patients with impaired immune systems, as seen with HIV/AIDS, advanced diabetes, drug abuse, or in the region of any prostheses. Clinicians should avoid entering the joint space or capsule with the needle. Lymph edema should be avoided when needling as there is a significantly increased risk of infections. To avoid infection practicing therapist must always wear gloves, and should always use sterile disposable needles, and must discard the used needles or oxidized needle in the bin only.

- Pneumothorax
  When needling around the thoracic region patients should be warned of the rare possibility of a pneumothorax. Care should be taken when needling upper trapezius and any other points over the thoracic region which could inadvertently create a pneumothorax. Where possible angle the needle away from the underlying lungs and/or needle over bone or cartilaginous tissue. Practitioners must have attended adequate training programs to needle in the thoracic region. The symptoms and signs of a pneumothorax may include shortness of breath on exertion, chest pain, dry cough, and decreased breath sounds on auscultation.

Such symptoms will commonly occur when the patient is walking away from the clinic. These symptoms may not occur until several hours after the treatment and patients need to be cautioned of this especially if they are going to be exposed to marked alterations in altitude such as flying or scuba diving. If a pneumothorax is suspected then the patient must be sent urgently for an x-ray and medical management.

- Needle stick injury

  Wash well around the site of penetration, encourage bleeding and have blood tests for hepatitis b and c and HIV/AIDS. The patient may also be requested to have the same blood analysis performed. If the patient is HIV positive, therapist should urgently seek medical advice. Practitioners should consider vaccinations for hepatitis b. Only therapists trained in dry needling techniques are permitted to remove needles from a patient. Clinicians should account for all needles and ensure adequate disposal into the sharps container. Keep the sharps container within easy reach of the treatment area, and do not overfill the box. Avoid rushing, interruptions during the treatment and do not needle when tired. Gloves should be worn though they may not fully protect against a needle stick injury, they may offer some level of protection, especially from contact with blood and bodily fluids. The risk of needle stick injury may extend to patients, patient family members, visitors, and other staff from a lost or forgotten needle and clinicians should ensure all needles are accounted for, safely discarded and that workstation design and access minimizes risk to third parties.

- Forgotten needles –

  To avoid this event best way is to count the number of needles therapist is inserting and count again while removing the needle. Secondary choose a path or an order of inserting the needles and follow the same path while removing them.

- Injury to internal organs:

  With dry needling an injury of an internal organ can be caused by the needle. A hematoma can be caused or an injury to the gastrointestinal tract which can lead to a serious intra-abdominal infection. The individual symptoms are very variable. Bleeding can cause damage to organs or shock. Signs for shock are tachycardia, decreased blood pressure, collapse of the throat veins, thirst, reduced micturition, flat breathing followed by reduced consciousness. Perforation of hollow organs and emission of gastrointestinal content can lead to peritonitis with sepsis, which expresses itself with abdominal pain, a tight abdominal wall and a high temperature. If a heavier relevant bleeding is suspected the patient must be referred to an emergency unit. Small hematomas without signs of shock can be analyzed through Ultrasound or MRI. In both cases medical advice should be called. This refers especially if there is suspicion of perforation of hollow organs (gastrointestinal tract or bladder).

- Vegetative reactions –

  This includes sudden change in blood pressure, pulse, respiratory rate, cold hand, muscle cramps, anxiety, agitations etc. In this state therapist must try to calm the patient as much as possible, stop dry needling and medical help is sought.

CHAPTER 3 – TRIGGER POINT DRY NEEDLING (UPPER QUARTER)

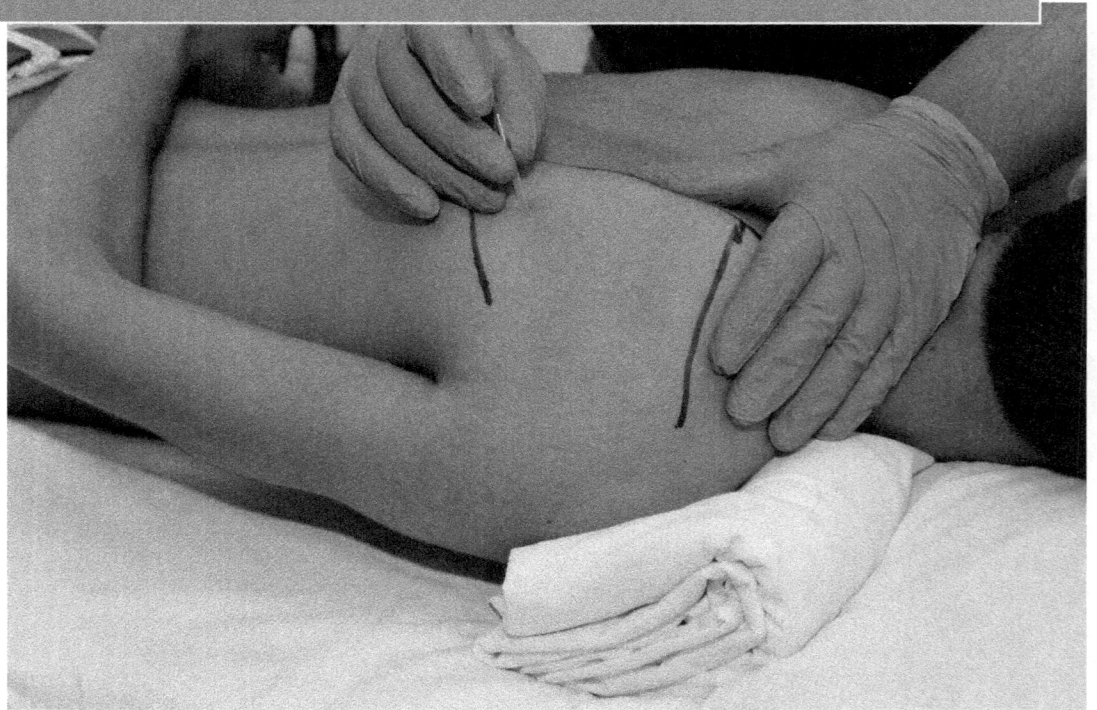

Supraspinatus

Basic Anatomy
Origin:
1. Supraspinous fossa,
2. Muscle fascia.

Insertion: Upper most of three facets of the greater tubercle of humerus.
Innervations: Suprascapular nerve, C5, 6.
Blood supply: Suprascapular artery.
Function:
1. Abduction of arm (first 15-20°),
2. Stabilizes glenohumeral joint.

Common sites of TrP & Referral pain: Refer to Figure 1.

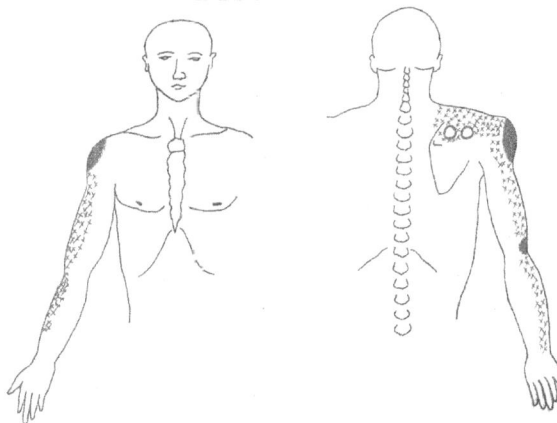

Figure 1: Referral pain pattern of TrP

Procedure
Patient position: Prone
Palpation:
1. **Bony landmarks-** Spine of Scapula
2. **Grip-** Flat

Technique: Deep Dry Needling
Needle size selection: 0.25mm X 25mm

Needle insertion: The trigger point is palpated for the supraspinatus muscle and the treatment area is cleaned properly. Needle is tapped into the skin at right angle and then angled laterally downwards towards acromion and spine of scapula.

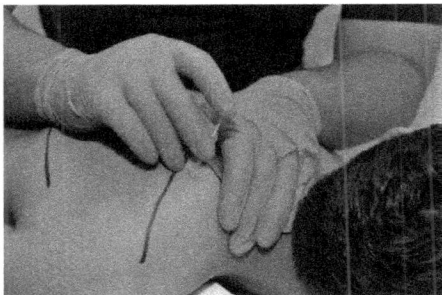

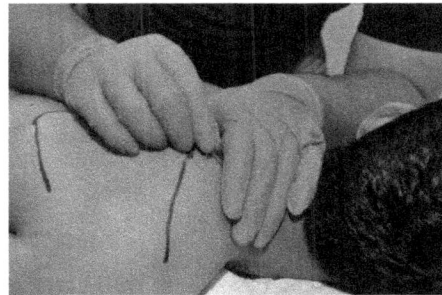

Figure 2: Dry Needling technique of Supraspinatus muscle TrP

Infraspinatus

Basic Anatomy
Origin:

1. Infraspinous fossa,
2. Muscle fascia.

Insertion: Middle facet of greater tubercle of humerus.
Innervations: Suprascapular nerve, C5, 6.
Blood supply: Suprascapular and circumflex scapular arteries.
Function:

1. External rotation of the humerus,
2. Stabilizes the glenohumeral joint.

Common sites of TrP & Referral pain: Refer to Figure 3.

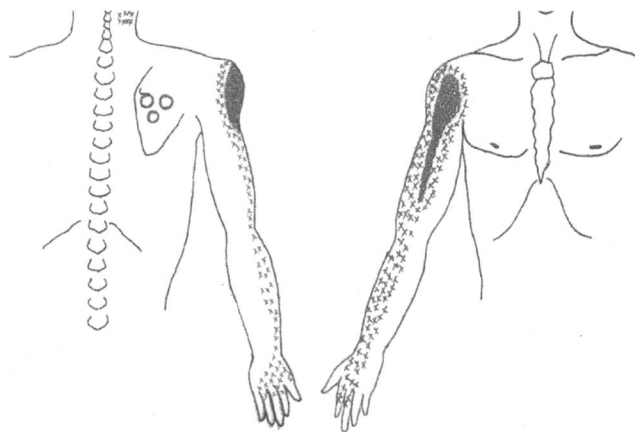

Figure 3: Referral pain pattern of TrP

Procedure
Patient position: Prone
Palpation:

1. **Bony landmarks-** Medial border of Scapula
2. **Grip-** Flat

Technique: Deep Dry Needling
Needle size selection: 0.25mm X 25mm

Needle insertion: The trigger point is palpated for the Infraspinatus muscle and the treatment area is cleaned properly. Needle is tapped into the skin at right angle and then angled superior-lateral towards the spine of scapula to cover the maximum area of muscle.

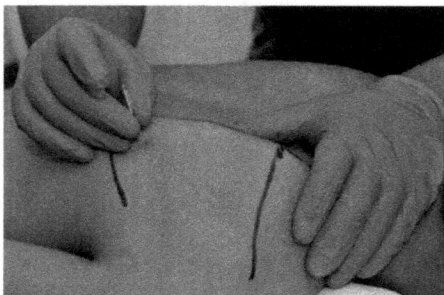

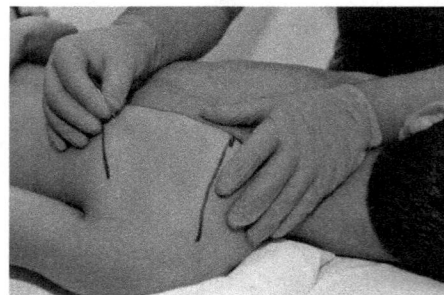

Figure 4: Dry Needling technique of Infraspinatus muscle TrP

Rhomboid Major and Rhomboid Minor

Basic Anatomy

Origin:

1. Rhomboid major- Sp nous processes of the T2 to T5 vertebrae.
2. Rhomboid minor-
    - Arises from the inferior border of the nuchal ligament,
    - From the spinous processes of the seventh cervical and first thoracic vertebrae,
    - And from the intervening supraspinous ligaments.

Insertion:

1. Rhomboid major-
    - Medial border of the scapula,
    - Inferior to the insertion of rhomboid minor muscle.
2. Rhomboid minor- Medial border of the scapula at the level of the scapular spine.

Innervations:

Rhomboid major and Rhomboid minor-Dorsal scapular nerve (C4 and C5).

Blood supply:

Rhomboid major and Rhomboid minor-Dorsal scapular artery.

Function:

Rhomboid major-
- Retracts the scapula and,
- Rotates the scapula to depress the glenoid cavity,
- It also fixes the scapula to the thoracic wall.

Rhomboid minor-
- Retracts and rotates scapula,
- Fixes scapula to thoracic wall.

Common sites of TrP & Referral pain: Refer to Figure 5.

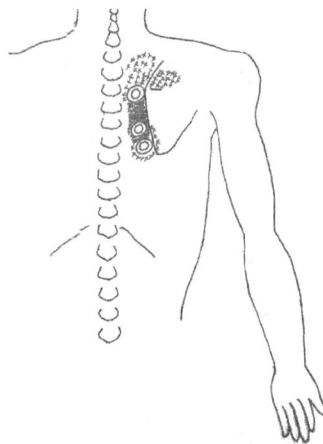

Figure 5: Referral pain pattern of TrP

Procedure

Patient position: Prone

Palpation:

1. **Bony landmarks-** Medial border of Scapula
2. **Grip-** Flat

Technique: Deep Dry Needling

Needle size selection: 0.25mm X 25mm

Needle insertion:
- Needle is tapped into the skin at right angle towards the medial border of scapula aimed towards the insertion of muscle. (Fig: 6)

- A smaller needle preferably 0.25 X 13mm needle is tapped into the skin while two fingers holding the trigger point, managing to keep it over the rib to avoid internal organ injury. The needle is then inserted at 45degree angle to treat the trigger point.(Fig: 7)

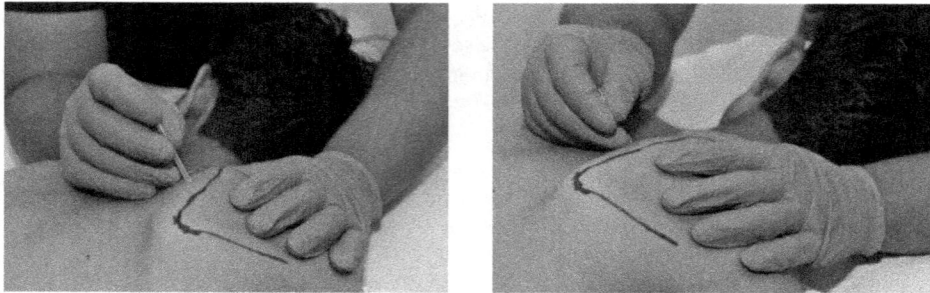

Figure 6: Dry Needling technique of Rhomboid muscle TrP (Attachment)

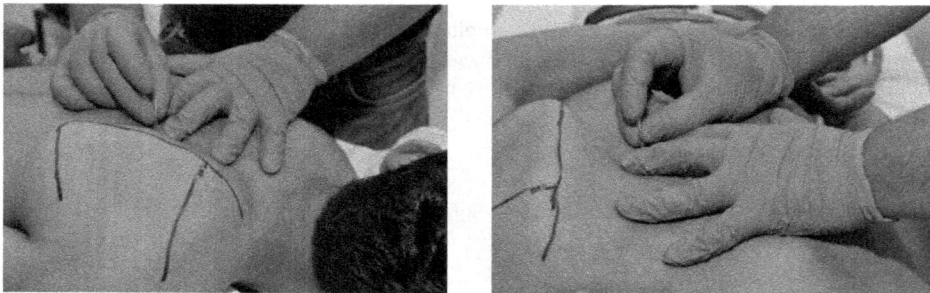

Figure 7: Dry Needling technique of Rhomboid muscle TrP (Belly)

Latissimus Dorsi

Basic Anatomy
Origin:

1. Spinous process of T7-L5, Thoracolumbar fascia,
2. Inferior angle of scapula,
3. Iliac crest,
4. Lower 3 or 4 Ribs.

Insertion: Lateral lip of the intertubercular groove of humerus.
Innervations: Thoracodorsal nerve, C6,7. 8.
Blood supply: Thoracodorsal branch of the subscapular artery.
Function:

1. Adduction& medial rotation of the humerus,
2. Extension from flexed position,
3. Downward rotation of the scapula.

Common sites of TrP & Referral pain: Refer to Figure 8.

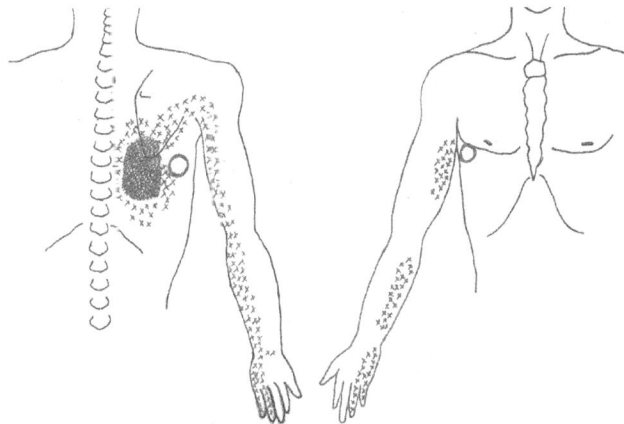

Figure 8: Referral pain pattern of TrP

Procedure
Patient position: Prone
Palpation:

1. **Bony landmarks-** Lateral border of Scapula
2. **Grip-** Pincer

Technique: Deep Dry Needling
Needle size selection: 0.25mm X 25mm

Needle insertion: Needle is tapped into the skin at right angle while one hand is holding the bulk of muscle with pincer grip. Needle is the guided into the muscle to treat the trigger point. Precautions are taken not to manipulate the needle towards the rib cage.

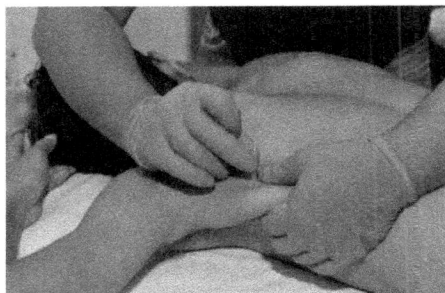

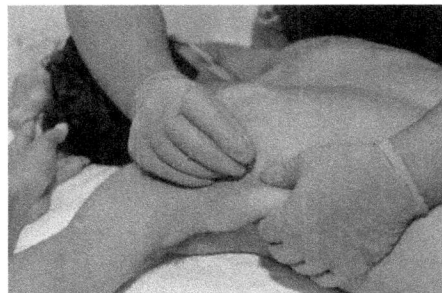

Figure 9: Dry Needling technique of Latissimus Dorsi muscle TrP

Upper Trapezius

Basic Anatomy

Origin:
1. External occipital protuberance,
2. Along the medial sides of the superior nuchal line,
3. Ligamentum nuchae (surrounding the cervical spinous processes),
4. Spinous processes of C1-T12.

Insertion:
1. Posterior, lateral 1/3 of clavicle,
2. Acromion process,
3. Superior spine of scapula.

Innervations:
1. Spinal Accessory (XI) (efferent or motor fibers),
2. Ventral ramii of C3 & C4 (afferent or sensory fibers).

Blood supply: Superficial cervical artery.

Function:
1. Elevates scapula,
2. Upward rotation of the scapula (upper fibers),
3. Downward rotation of the scapula (lower fibers),
4. Retracts scapula.

Common sites of TrP & Referral pain: Refer to Figure 10.

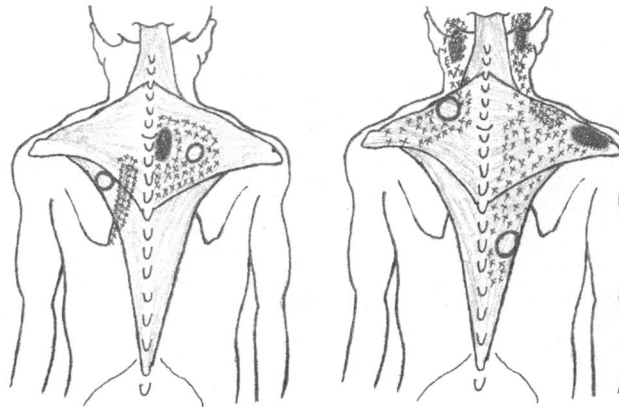

Figure 10: Referral pain pattern of TrP

Procedure

Patient position: Prone

Palpation:
1. **Bony landmarks-** Acromion process
2. **Grip-** Pincer Grip

Technique: Deep Dry Needling

Needle size selection: 0.25mm X 25mm / 0.25mm X 40mm

Caution: Caution must be taken while needling the upper trapezius as it lies near to apex of lung.

Needle insertion: The muscle is grasped with one hand with pincer grip and carefully lifted away to clear the treatment area. The needle is tapped at right angle to the belly of muscle. The needle is then manipulated in the muscle belly ensuring it reaches the trigger point to get a localized twitch response.

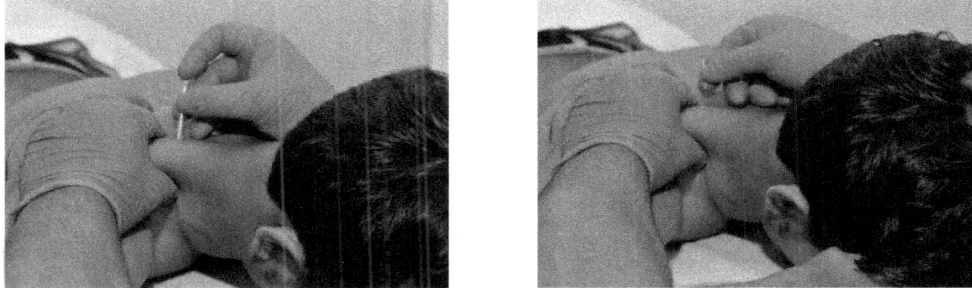

Figure 11: Dry Needling technique of Upper Trapezius muscle TrP

Teres Major

Basic Anatomy

Origin: Dorsal surface of the inferior angle of the scapula,

Insertion: Medial lip of the intertubercular sulcus of the humerus.

Innervations: Lower Sub scapular Nerve, C5, 6.

Blood supply: Subscapular and circumflex scapular arteries.

Function:

1. Assists in adduction of arm,
2. Assists in medial rotation of arm,
3. Assists in extension from a flexed position.

Common sites of TrP & Referral pain: Refer to Figure 12.

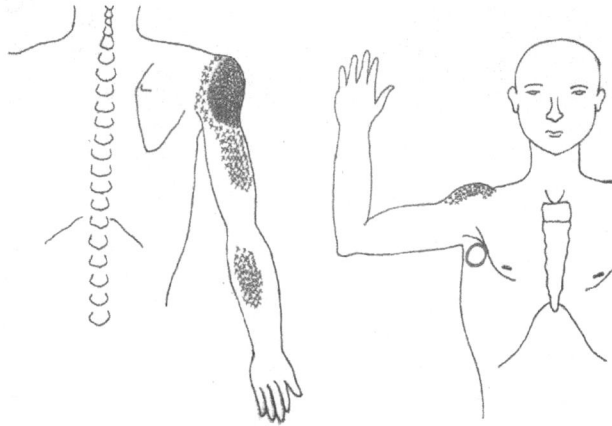

Figure 12: Referral pain pattern of TrP

Procedure

Patient position: Supine with arm abducted

Palpation:

1. **Bony landmarks-** Rib Cage
2. **Grip-** Pincer Grip

Technique: Deep Dry Needling

Needle size selection: 0.25mm X 25mm / 0.25mm X 40mm

Caution: Caution must be taken to avoid directing needle towards the rig cage.

Needle insertion: The muscle is grasped with one hand with pincer grip and carefully lifted away from rib cage just below the axilla to clear the treatment area. The needle is tapped at right angle to the belly of muscle. The needle is then manipulated in the muscle belly ensuring it reaches the trigger point to get a localized twitch response.

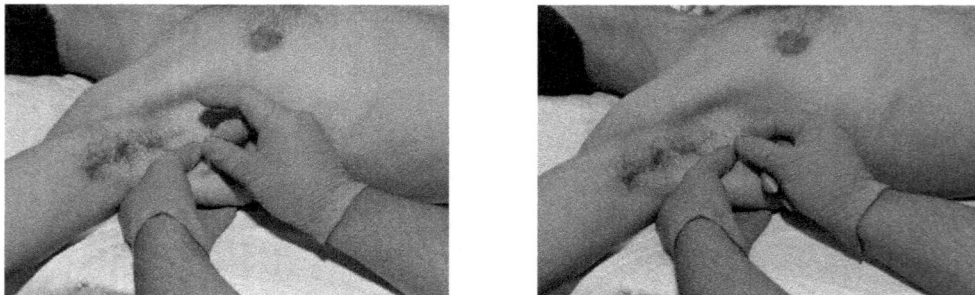

Figure 13: Dry Needling technique of Teres Major muscle TrP

Teres Minor

Basic Anatomy
Origin:.
- It arises from the dorsal surface of the axillary border of the scapula for the upper two-thirds of its extent,
- From two aponeurotic laminae, one of which separates it from the infraspinatus muscle, the other from the teres major muscle.

Insertion: Inferior facet of greater tubercle of the humerus.
Innervations: Axillary nerve.
Blood supply: Posterior circumflex humeral artery and the circumflex scapular artery.
Function: Laterally rotates the arm, stabilizes humerus.

Common sites of TrP & Referral pain: Refer to Figure 14.

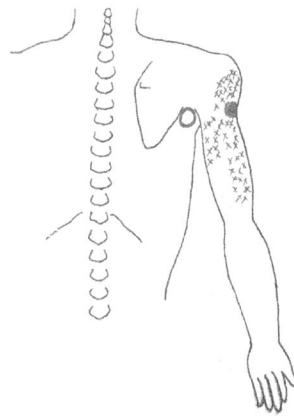

Figure 14: Referral pain pattern of TrP

Procedure
Patient position: Supine with arm abducted
Palpation:
1. **Bony landmarks-** Rib Cage
2. **Grip-** Pincer Grip

Technique: Deep Dry Needling
Needle size selection: 0.25mm X 25mm / 0.25mm X 40mm
Caution: Caution must be taken to avoid directing needle towards the rig cage.

Needle insertion: The muscle is grasped with one hand with pincer grip and carefully lifted away from rib cage just below the axilla to clear the treatment area. The needle is tapped at right angle to the belly of muscle. The needle is then manipulated in the muscle belly ensuring it reaches the trigger point to get a localized twitch response.

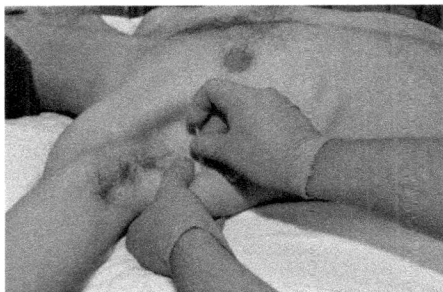

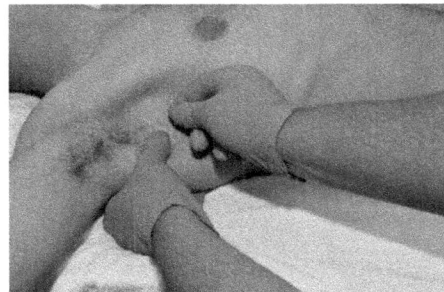

Figure 15: Dry Needling technique of Teres Minor muscle TrP

Subscapularis

Basic Anatomy
Origin: Subscapular fossa.
Insertion: Lesser tubercle of humerus.
Innervations: Upper subscapular nerve, lower subscapular nerve (C5, C6).
Blood supply: Subscapular artery.
Function: Internally (medially) rotates humerus; stabilizes shoulder.

Common sites of TrP & Referral pain: Refer to Figure 16.

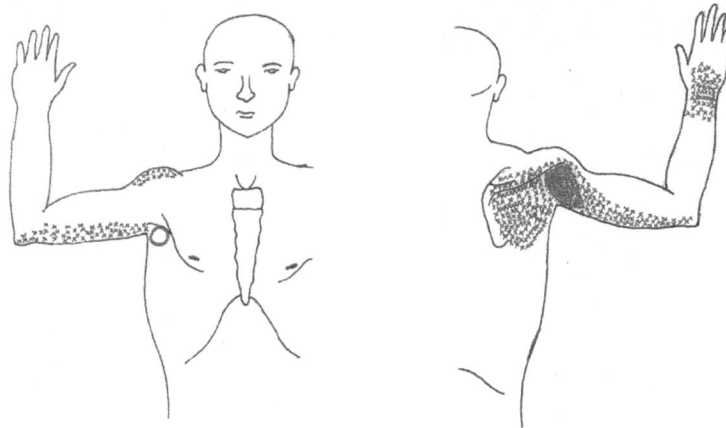

Figure 16: Referral pain pattern of TrP

Procedure
Patient position: Supine with arm abducted
Palpation:
1. **Bony landmarks-** lateral border of scapula and anterior surface of scapula
2. **Grip-** Flat

Technique: Deep Dry Needling
Needle size selection: 0.25mm X 25mm / 0.25mm X 40mm
Caution: Caution must be taken to avoid directing needle towards the rig cage.

Needle insertion: The muscle lies on the anterior surface of scapula, the arm is 90 degree abducted and thumb is placed on the anterior surface of scapula pushing the scapula posteriorly. The needle is tapped at an angle of 45degree to the surface of scapula to ensure it enters the muscle, while the direction is away from rib cage. The needle is then manipulated in the muscle belly ensuring it reaches the trigger point to get a localized twitch response.

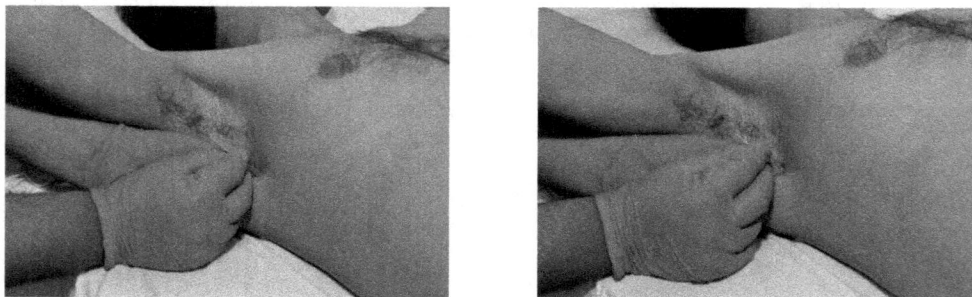

Figure 17: Dry Needling technique of Subscapularis muscle TrP

Levator Scapulae

Basic Anatomy

Origin: Transverse Processes of C1-C3 or C4.

Insertion: Superior angle of scapula toward the scapular spine.

Innervations:

1. Nerves off cervical plexus, C3,4,
2. Dorsal scapular nerve, C5.

Blood supply: Dorsal scapular artery.

Function:

1. Elevates the scapula,
2. Tilts its glenoid cavity inferiorly by rotating scapula.

Common sites of TrP & Referral pain: Refer to Figure 18.

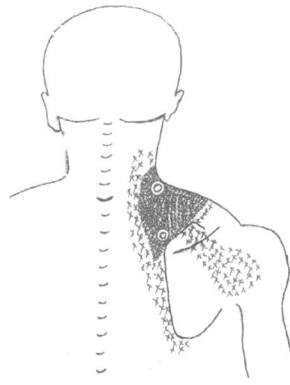

Figure 18: Referral pain pattern of TrP

Procedure

Patient position: Prone

Palpation:

1. **Bony landmarks-** Scapula superio- medial border
2. **Grip-** Flat Grip

Technique: Deep Dry Needling

Needle size selection: 0.25mm X 25mm

Needle insertion: Therapist keeps his fingers on the either side of the superio-medial border, ensuring the trigger point is between the fingers. The needle is tapped at right angle towards the border of the scapula. The needle is then manipulated in the muscle belly ensuring it reaches the trigger point to get a localized twitch response.

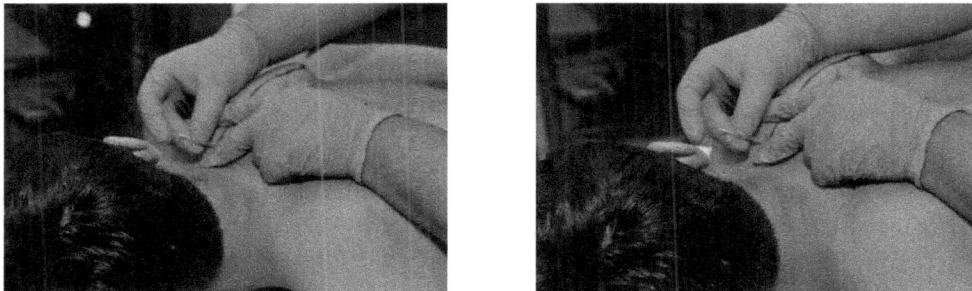

Figure 19: Dry Needling technique of Levator Scapulae muscle TrF

Deltoid

Basic Anatomy

Origin:

1. Lateral, anterior 1/3 of distal clavicle,
2. Lateral boarder of the acromion process,
3. Scapular spine.

Insertion: Deltoid tuberosity of humerus.

Innervations: Axillary nerve, C5.

Blood supply: Thoraco-acromial artery, anterior and posterior humeral circumflex artery.

Function:

1. Abducts arm,
2. Flexion and medial rotation (anterior portion),
3. Extension and lateral rotation (posterior portion).

Common sites of TrP & Referral pain: Refer to Figure 20.

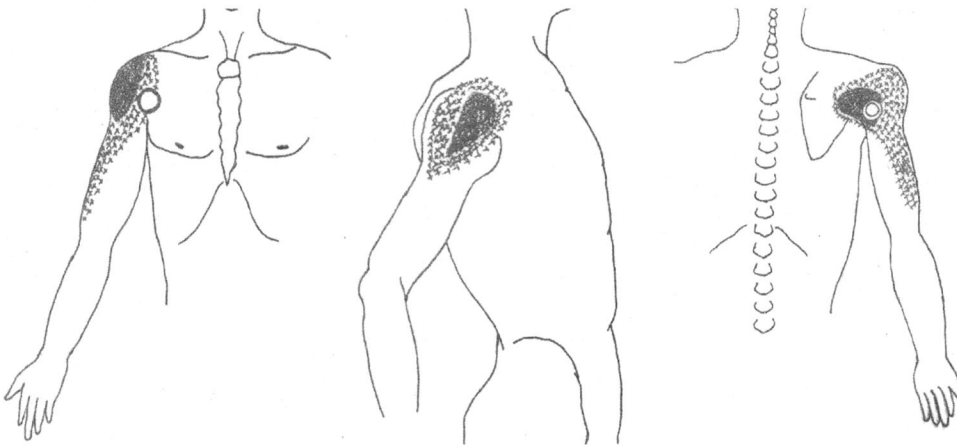

Figure 20: Referral pain pattern of TrP

Procedure

Patient position: Prone/ Supine

Palpation:

1. **Bony landmarks-** Deltoid tubrosity, Acromion process, Clavicle, Spine of Scapula
2. **Grip-** Flat Grip

Technique: Deep Dry Needling

Needle size selection: 0.25mm X 25mm / 0.25mm X 40mm

Caution: Caution must be taken to avoid injury to Axillary nerve.

Needle insertion:

1. The trigger point is palpated for the Deltoid Anterior fibers and the treatment area is cleaned properly. Needle is tapped into the skin at right angle and then angled laterally outwards.(Fig 21)
2. The trigger point is palpated for the Deltoid Middle fibers and the treatment area is cleaned properly. Needle is tapped into the skin at right angle and then angled Upwards.(Fig 22)
3. The trigger point is palpated for the Deltoid Posterior fibers and the treatment area is cleaned properly. Needle is tapped into the skin at right angle and then angled towards the trigger point.(Fig 23)

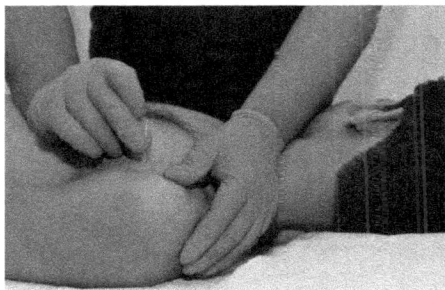

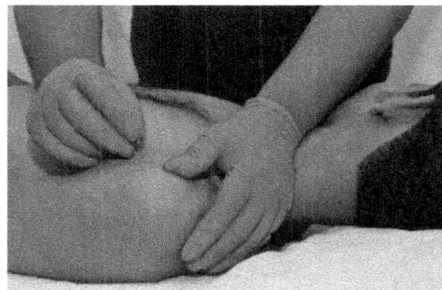

Figure 21: Dry Needling technique of Deltoid Anterior Fibers TrP

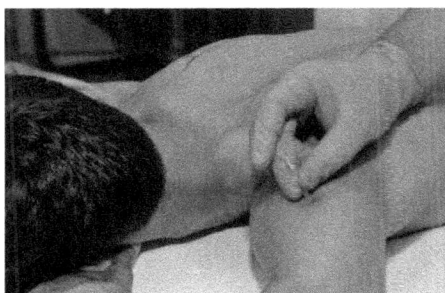

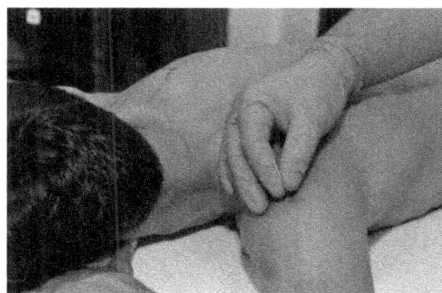

Figure 22: Dry Needling technique of Deltoid Middle Fibers TrP

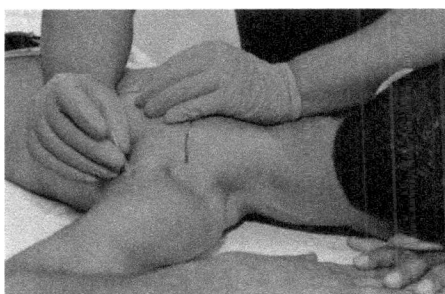

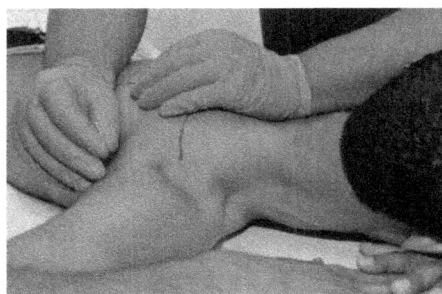

Figure 23: Dry Needling technique of Deltoid Posterior Fibers TrP

Biceps

Basic Anatomy
Origin:
- **Short head:** Coracoid process of the scapula,
- **Long head:** Supraglenoid tubercle.

Insertion: Radial tuberosity and bicipital aponeurosis into deep fascia on medial part of forearm.
Innervations: Musculocutaneous nerve (C5–C6).
Blood supply: Brachial artery.
Function: Flexes elbow and supinates forearm.

Common sites of TrP & Referral pain: Refer to Figure 24.

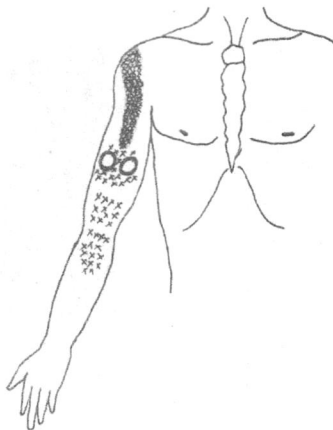

Figure 24: Referral pain pattern of TrP

Procedure
Patient position: Supine
Palpation:
1. **Bony landmarks-** Humerus
2. **Grip-** Pincer Grip

Technique: Deep Dry Needling
Needle size selection: 0.25mm X 25mm / 0.25mm X 40mm
Caution: Needling towards the shaft of humerus is avoided to prevent injury to brachial artery.

Needle insertion: The trigger point is palpated for the Biceps muscle and the treatment area is cleaned properly. Needle is tapped into the skin at right angle to muscle belly and then angled towards the trigger point.

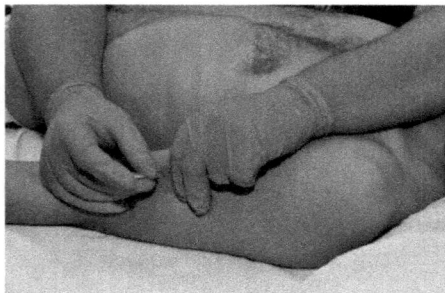

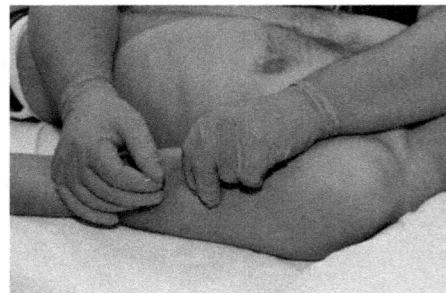

Figure 25: Dry Needling technique of Biceps Muscle TrP

Triceps

Basic Anatomy

Origin:

- **Long head:** Infra glenoid tubercle of scapula,
- **Lateral head:** Above the radial sulcus,
- **Medial head:** Below the radial sulcus.

Insertion: Olecranon process of ulna.

Innervations: Radial nerve and axillary nerve (long head).

Blood supply: Deep brachial artery.

Function: Extends forearm, long head extends shoulder.

Common sites of TrP & Referral pain: Refer to Figure 26.

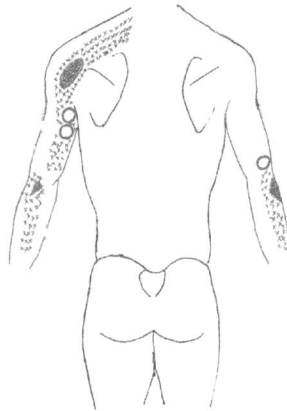

Figure 25: Referral pain pattern of TrP

Procedure

Patient position: Prone

Palpation:

1. **Bony landmarks-** Humerus
2. **Grip-** Pincer Grip

Technique: Deep Dry Needling

Needle size selection: 0.25mm X 25mm / 0.25mm X 40mm

Needle insertion: The trigger point is palpated for the Triceps muscle and the treatment area is cleaned properly. Needle is tapped into the skin at right angle to muscle belly and then angled towards the trigger point.

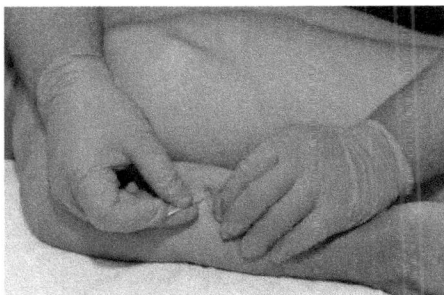

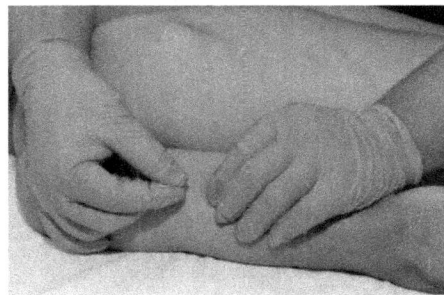

Figure 27: Dry Needling technique of Triceps Muscle TrP

Anconeus

Basic Anatomy

Origin: The posterior surface of the lateral epicondyle of the humerus.

Insertion: Ulna- lateral to the olecranon from where it extends down on the dorsal side of the bone.

Innervations: Radial nerve (C7,C8,T1).

Blood supply: Deep brachial artery, recurrent interosseous artery.

Function:

- It assists in extension of the forearm by partly blending in with the triceps,
- It also stabilizes the elbow during pronation and supination.
- Pulls slack out of the elbow joint capsule during extension to prevent impingement.

Common sites of TrP & Referral pain: Refer to Figure 28.

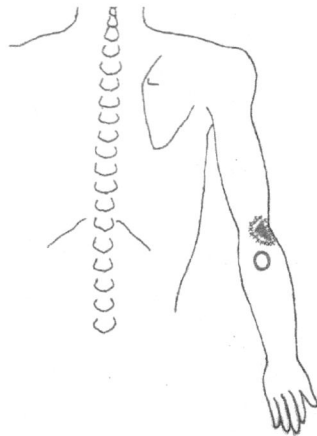

Figure 28: Referral pain pattern of TrP

Procedure

Patient position: Prone

Palpation:

1. **Bony landmarks-** Lateral Epicondyle
2. **Grip-** Flat Grip

Technique: Deep Dry Needling

Needle size selection: 0.25mm X 25mm

Needle insertion: The trigger point is palpated for the Anconeus muscle and the treatment area is cleaned properly. Needle is tapped into the skin at right angle to muscle belly and then angled towards the trigger point.

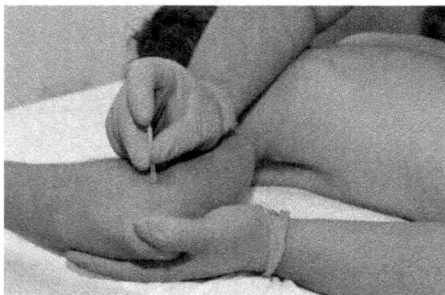

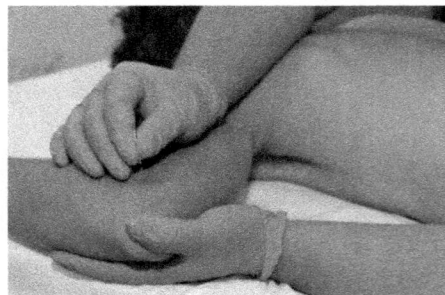

Figure 29: Dry Needling technique of Anconeus Muscle TrP

Brachialis

Basic Anatomy
Origin:
- From the lower half of the front of the humerus,
- Anterior surface of the humerus, particularly the distal half of this bone,
- It also arises from the intermuscular septa of the arm.

Insertion: Coronoid process and the tuberosity of the ulna.
Innervations: Musculocutaneous nerve (C5, C6).
Blood supply: Radial recurrent artery.
Function: Flexion at elbow joint.

Common sites of TrP & Referral pain: Refer to Figure 30.

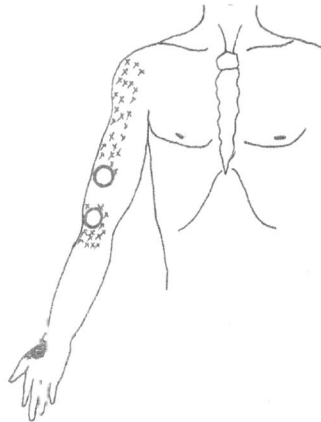

Figure 30: Referral pain pattern of TrP

Patient position: Supine
Palpation:
1. **Bony landmarks-** Humerus
2. **Grip-** Pincer Grip

Technique: Deep Dry Needling
Needle size selection: 0.25mm X 25mm

Needle insertion: The biceps muscle is grasped with one hand with pincer grip and carefully lifted to clear the treatment area for Brachialis. The needle is tapped at right angle just below the biceps belly to reach brachialis. The needle is then manipulated in the muscle belly ensuring it reaches the trigger point to get a localized twitch response.

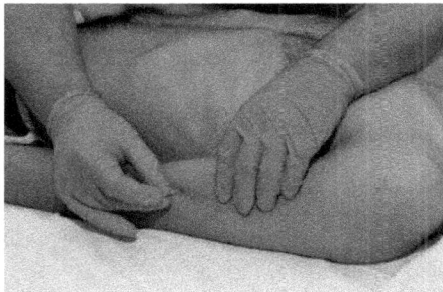

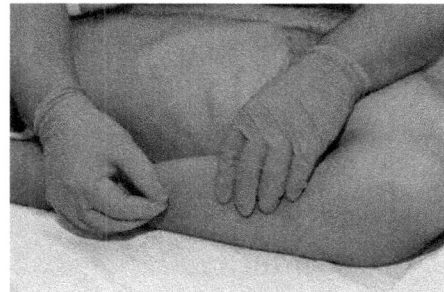

Figure 31: Dry Needling technique of Brachialis Muscle TrP

Brachioradialis

Basic Anatomy
Origin: Lateral supracondylar ridge of the humerus.
Insertion: Distal radius (Radial styloid process).
Innervations: Radial nerve.
Blood supply: Radial recurrent artery.
Function: Flexion of Elbow.

Common sites of TrP & Referral pain: Refer to Figure 32.

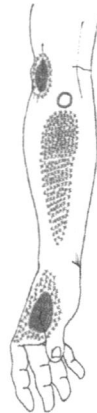

Figure 32: Referral pain pattern of TrP

Procedure
Patient position: Sitting with forearm Supported
Palpation:
1. **Bony landmarks-** Lateral Epicondyle of Humerus
2. **Grip-** Pincer Grip

Technique: Deep Dry Needling
Needle size selection: 0.25mm X 25mm

Needle insertion: The Brachioradialis muscle is grasped with one hand with pincer grip and carefully lifted to clear the treatment area. The needle is tapped at right angle to muscle belly. The needle is then manipulated in the muscle belly ensuring it reaches the trigger point to get a localized twitch response.

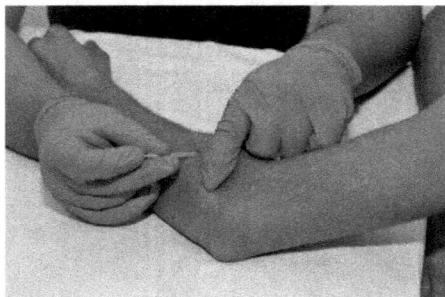

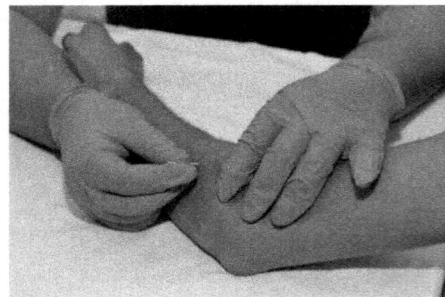

Figure 33: Dry Needling technique of Brachioradialis Muscle TrP

Supinator

Basic Anatomy
Origin:
- Lateral epicondyle of humerus,
- Supinator crest of ulna,
- Radial collateral ligament,
- Annular ligament.

Insertion: Lateral proximal radial shaft.
Innervations: Posterior interosseous nerve, (a continuation of the deep branch of the radial nerve).
Blood supply: Radial recurrent artery.
Function: .Supinates forearm

Common sites of TrP & Referral pain: Refer to Figure 34.

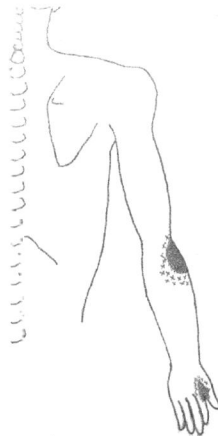

Figure 34: Referral pain pattern of TrP

Procedure
Patient position: Sitting with forearm Supported
Palpation:
1. **Bony landmarks-** Lateral epicondyle
2. **Grip-** Flat Grip

Technique: Deep Dry Needling
Needle size selection: 0.25mm X 25mm / 0.25mm X 40mm

Needle insertion: The trigger point is palpated for the Supinator muscle and the treatment area is cleaned properly. Needle is tapped into the skin at right angle and then angled laterally downwards towards muscle belly to elicit a twitch response.

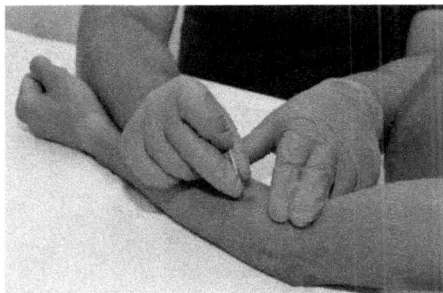

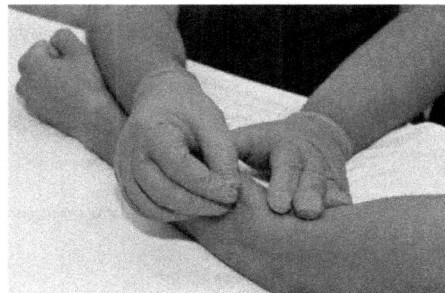

Figure 35: Dry Needling technique of Supinator Muscle TrP

Extensor Carpi Radialis Brevis

Basic Anatomy

Origin: Humerus at the anterior of lateral epicondyle (common extensor tendon).

Insertion: Posterior base of the 3rd metacarpal.

Innervations: Deep branch of the radial nerve.

Blood supply: Radial artery.

Function: Extensor and abductor of the hand at the wrist joint.

Common sites of TrP & Referral pain: Refer to Figure 36.

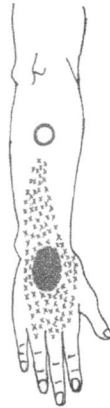

Figure 36: Referral pain pattern of TrP

Procedure

Patient position: Sitting with forearm Supported

Palpation:

1. **Bony landmarks-** Lateral epicondyle
2. **Grip-** Flat Grip

Technique: Deep Dry Needling

Needle size selection: 0.25mm X 25mm / 0.25mm X 40mm

Needle insertion: The trigger point is palpated for the ECRB muscle and the treatment area is cleaned properly. Needle is tapped into the skin at right angle, directed towards the radius and then manipulated towards muscle belly to elicit a twitch response.

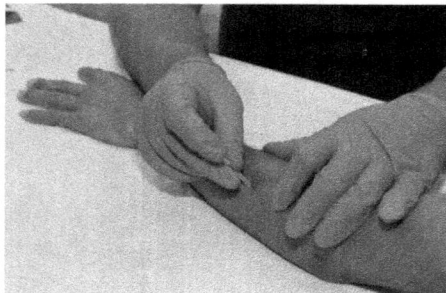

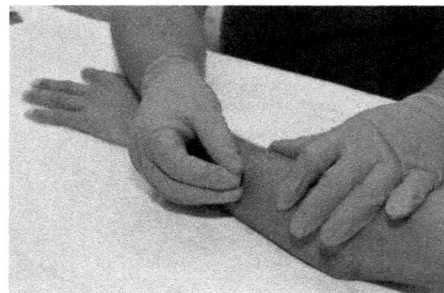

Figure 37: Dry Needling technique of Extensor Carpi Radialis Brevis Muscle TrP

Extensor Digitorum

Basic Anatomy
Origin:
- It arises from the lateral epicondyle of the humerus (common extensor tendon),
- From the intermuscular septa , the adjacent muscles, and from the antebrachial fascia.

Insertion: Extensor expansion of middle and distal phalanges of the 2nd, 3rd, 4th, and 5th fingers.
Innervations: Radial nerve.
Blood supply: Posterior interosseous artery.
Function:
- The extensor digitorum communis extends the phalanges, the wrist, and finally the elbow.
- It acts principally on the proximal phalanges, the middle and terminal phalanges being extended mainly by the interossei and lumbricales.
- It tends to separate the fingers as it extends them.

Common sites of TrP & Referral pain: Refer to Figure 38.

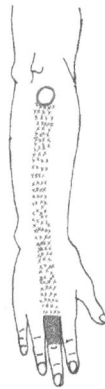

Figure 38: Referral pain pattern of TrP

Procedure
Patient position: Sitting with forearm Supported
Palpation:
1. **Bony landmarks-** Lateral epicondyle
2. **Grip-** Flat Grip

Technique: Deep Dry Needling
Needle size selection: 0.25mm X 25mm / 0.25mm X 40mm

Needle insertion: The trigger point is palpated for the Extensor Digitorum muscle and the treatment area is cleaned properly. Needle is tapped into the skin at right angle, directed towards the muscle belly to elicit a twitch response.

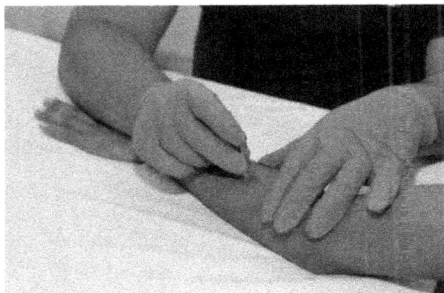

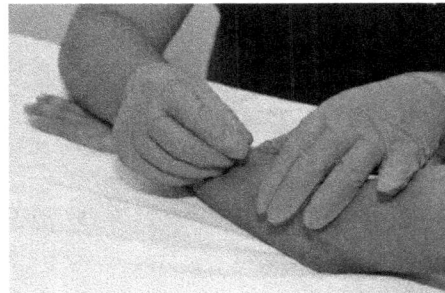

Figure 39: Dry Needling technique of Extensor Digitorum Muscle TrP

Extensor Carpi Ulnaris

Basic Anatomy
Origin: Its arise from the lateral epicondyle of the humerus and the posterior border of ulna.
Insertion: Base of the 5th metacarpal.
Innervations: Posterior interosseous nerve (C7 and C8), the continuation of the deep branch of the radial nerve.
Blood supply: Ulnar artery.
Function: Extension and adduction of the wrist.

Common sites of TrP & Referral pain: Refer to Figure 40.

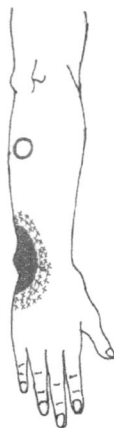

Figure 40: Referral pain pattern of TrP

Procedure
Patient position: Sitting with forearm Supported
Palpation:
1. **Bony landmarks-** Lateral epicondyle of humerus, Ulna
2. **Grip-** Flat Grip

Technique: Deep Dry Needling
Needle size selection: 0.25mm X 25mm / 0.25mm X 40mm

Needle insertion: The trigger point is palpated for the ECU muscle and the treatment area is cleaned properly. Needle is tapped into the skin at right angle, directed medially and then manipulated towards muscle belly to elicit a twitch response.

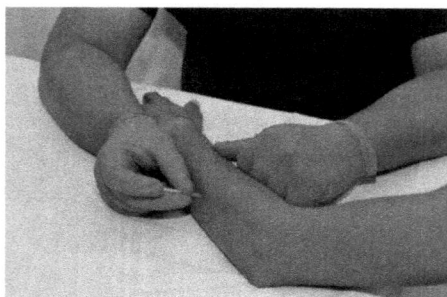

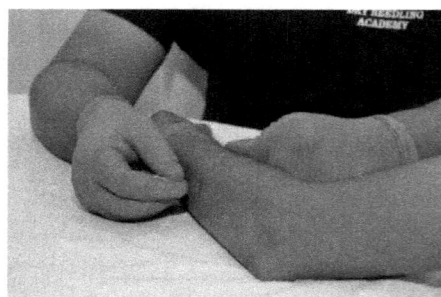

Figure 41: Dry Needling technique of Extensor Carpi Ulnaris Muscle TrP

Pronator Teres

Basic Anatomy
Origin:
- Humeral head: medial epicondyle of humerus (common flexor tendon),
- Ulnar head: coronoid process of ulna.

Insertion: Middle of the lateral surface of the body of the radius.
Innervations: Median nerve.
Blood supply: Ulnar artery and radial artery.
Function: Pronation of forearm, flexes elbow.

Common sites of TrP & Referral pain: Refer to Figure 42.

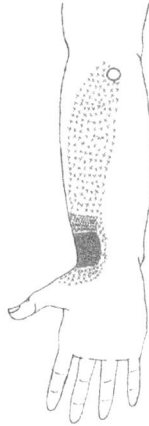

Figure 42: Referral pain pattern of TrP

Procedure
Patient position: Sitting with forearm Supported
Palpation:
1. **Bony landmarks-** Medial epicondyle of humerus
2. **Grip-** Flat Grip

Technique: Deep Dry Needling
Needle size selection: 0.25mm X 25mm / 0.25mm X 40mm

Needle insertion: The trigger point is palpated for the Pronator Teres muscle and the treatment area is cleaned properly. Needle is tapped into the skin at right angle, directed towards the muscle belly to elicit a twitch response.

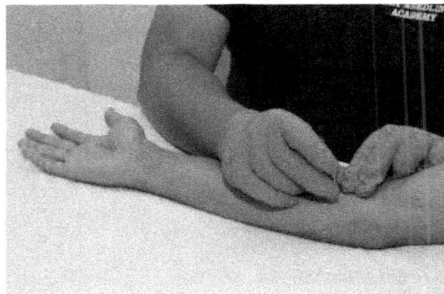

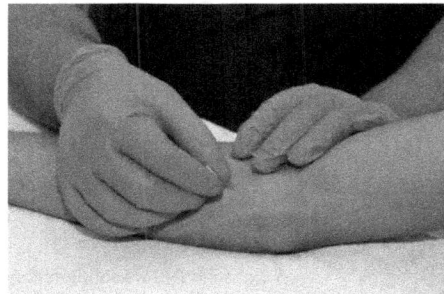

Figure 43: Dry Needling technique of Pronator Teres Muscle TrP

Flexor Carpi Radialis

Basic Anatomy
Origin: Medial condyle of the humerus.
Insertion: Base of the 2nd and 3rd metacarpal bone.
Innervations: Median nerve.
Blood supply: Ulnar artery.
Function: Flexion and abduction of wrist.

Common sites of TrP & Referral pain: Refer to Figure 44.

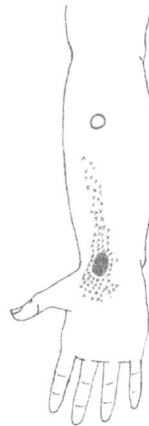

Figure 44: Referral pain pattern of TrP

Procedure
Patient position: Sitting with forearm Supported
Palpation:
1. **Bony landmarks-** Medial epicondyle
2. **Grip-** Flat Grip

Technique: Deep Dry Needling
Needle size selection: 0.25mm X 25mm / 0.25mm X 40mm

Needle insertion: The trigger point is palpated for the FCR muscle and the treatment area is cleaned properly. Needle is tapped into the skin at right angle, directed towards the muscle belly to elicit a twitch response.

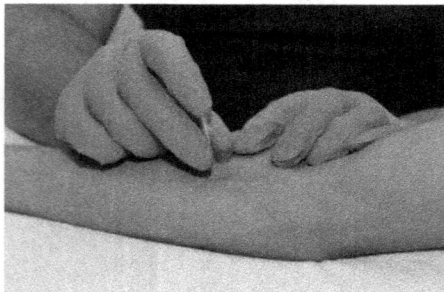

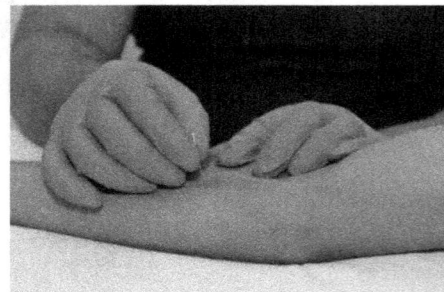

Figure 45: Dry Needling technique of Flexor Carpi Radialis Muscle TrP

Flexor Digitorum Profundus and Superficialis

Basic Anatomy
Origin:
- Flexor digitorum profundus: Upper 3/4 of the volar and medial surfaces of the body of the ulna, interosseous membrane and deep fascia of the forearm.
- Flexor digitorum superficialis: Medial epicondyle of the humerus (common flexor tendon) as well as parts of the radius and ulna.

Insertion:
- Flexor digitorum profundus: Base of the distal phalanges of the fingers.
- Flexor digitorum superficialis: Anterior margins on the bases of the middle phalanges of four fingers.

Innervations:
- Flexor digitorum profundus: Median (anterior interosseous),muscular branches of ulnar.
- Flexor digitorum superficialis: Median nerve (C7, C8, T1).

Blood supply:
- Flexor digitorum profundus: Anterior interosseous artery.
- Flexor digitorum superficialis: Ulnar artery.

Function:
- Flexor digitorum profundus: Flex hand and interphalangeal joints.
- Flexor digitorum superficialis: Flexion of the middle phalanges of the fingers at the proximal interphalangeal joints, however under continued action it also flexes the metacarpo-phalangeal joints and wrist joint.

Common sites of TrP & Referral pain: Refer to Figure 46.

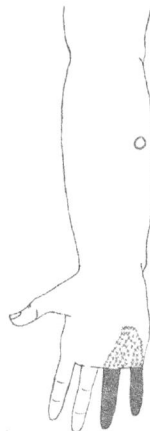

Figure 46: Referral pain pattern of TrP

Procedure
Patient position: Sitting with forearm Supported
Palpation:
1. **Bony landmarks-** Medial Epicondyle
2. **Grip-** Flat Grip

Technique: Deep Dry Needling
Needle size selection: 0.25mm X 25mm / 0.25mm X 40mm

Needle insertion: The trigger point is palpated for the Flexor Digitorum muscle and the treatment area is cleaned properly. Needle is tapped into the skin at right angle, directed towards the muscle belly to elicit a twitch response.

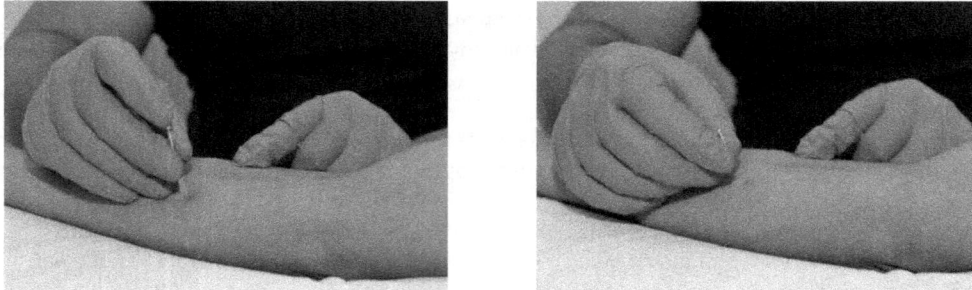

Figure 47: Dry Needling technique of Flexor Digitorum Muscle TrP

Adductor Pollicis

Basic Anatomy
Origin:
- Transverse head: anterior body of the third metacarpal
- Oblique head: bases of the second and the third metacarpals and the adjacent trapezoid and capitate bones.

Insertion: Medial side of the base of the proximal phalanx of the thumb and the ulnar sesamoid.
Innervations: Deep branch of the ulnar nerve (T1).
Blood supply: Deep palmar arch.
Function:
- Adducts the thumb at the carpo-metacarpal joint
- It can also bring the thumb to the side of the palm and index finger

Common sites of TrP & Referral pain: Refer to Figure 48.

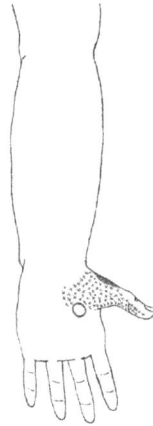

Figure 48: Referral pain pattern of TrP

Procedure
Patient position: Sitting with wrist supported
Palpation:
1. **Bony landmarks-** First and second metacarpals
2. **Grip-** Flat Grip

Technique: Deep Dry Needling
Needle size selection: 0.25mm X 25mm / 0.25mm X 40mm

Needle insertion: The trigger point is palpated for the Adductor Pollicis muscle and the treatment area is cleaned properly. Needle is tapped into the skin at right angle, directed towards the muscle belly to elicit a twitch response.

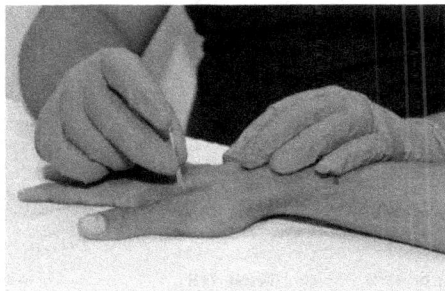

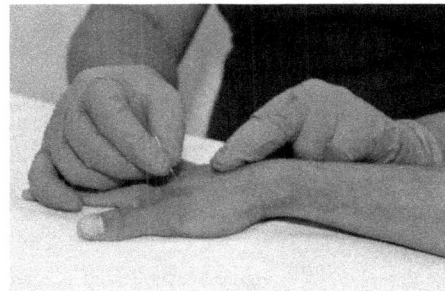

Figure 49: Dry Needling technique of Adductor Pollicis Muscle TrP

Opponens Pollicis

Basic Anatomy
Origin:
- From the flexor retinaculum of the hand and,
- The tubercle of the trapezium.

Insertion: Metacarpal bone of the thumb on its radial side.
Innervations: Recurrent branch of the median nerve.
Blood supply: Superficial palmar arch.
Function: Flexion of the thumb's metacarpal at the first carpometacarpal joint, which aids in opposition of the thumb.

Common sites of TrP & Referral pain: Refer to Figure 50.

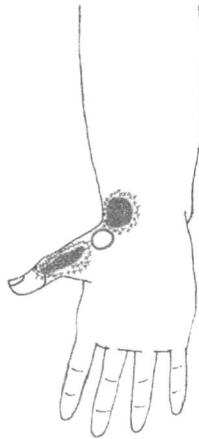

Figure 50: Referral pain pattern of TrP

Procedure
Patient position: Sitting with wrist supported
Palpation:
1. **Bony landmarks-** First Metacarpal
2. **Grip-** Flat Grip

Technique: Deep Dry Needling
Needle size selection: 0.25mm X 25mm / 0.25mm X 40mm

Needle insertion: The trigger point is palpated for the Opponens Pollicis muscle and the treatment area is cleaned properly. Needle is tapped into the skin at right angle, directed towards the muscle belly to elicit a twitch response.

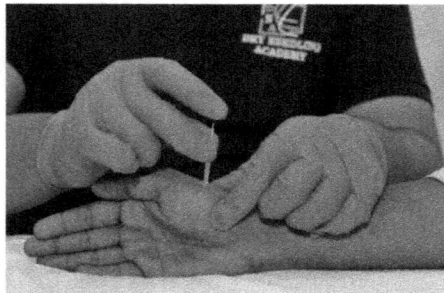

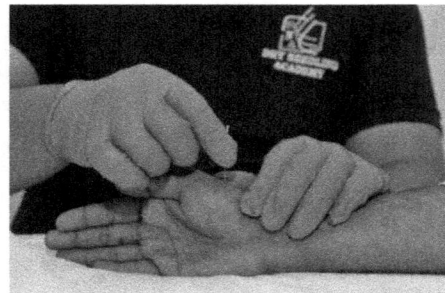

Figure 51: Dry Needling technique of Opponens Pollicis Muscle TrP

Abductor Pollicis Brevis

Basic Anatomy

Origin:
- Transverse carpal ligament,
- The tubercle of scaphoid and
- Tubercle of the trapezium.

Insertion:
- Radial base of proximal phalanx of thumb and,
- The capsule of the metacarpo-phalangeal joint.

Innervations: Recurrent branch of the median nerve C8/T1.

Blood supply: Superficial palmar arch.

Function:
- Abduction of the thumb by acting across the carpometacarpal joint and the metacarpo-phalangeal joint.
- It also assists in opposition and extension of the thumb.

Common sites of TrP & Referral pain: Refer to Figure 52.

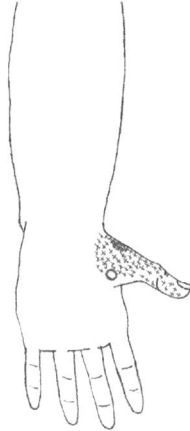

Figure 52: Referral pain pattern of TrP

Procedure

Patient position: Sitting with wrist supported

Palpation:
1. **Bony landmarks-** First Metacarpal
2. **Grip-** Flat Grip

Technique: Deep Dry Needling

Needle size selection: 0.25mm X 25mm / 0.25mm X 40mm

Needle insertion: The trigger point is palpated for the Abductor Pollicis Brevis muscle and the treatment area is cleaned properly. Needle is tapped into the skin at right angle, directed towards the muscle belly to elicit a twitch response.

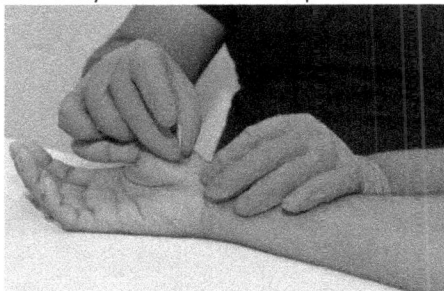

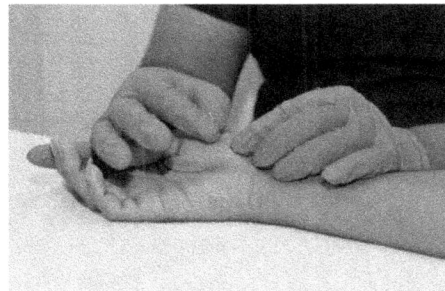

Figure 53: Dry Needling technique of Abductor Pollicis Brevis Muscle TrP

Dorsal Interossei

Basic Anatomy

Origin: Dorsal 1-4: adjacent sides of 2 metacarpals

Insertion: Dorsal 1-4: extensor expansions and base of proximal phalanges

Innervations: Deep branch of ulnar nerve.

Blood supply: Dorsal and palmar metacarpal artery.

Function: Abduct the finger.

Common sites of TrP & Referral pain: Refer to Figure 54.

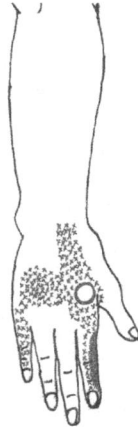

Figure 54: Referral pain pattern of TrP

Procedure

Patient position: Sitting with forearm & wrist supported.

Palpation:

1. **Bony landmarks-** Metacarpal shaft
2. **Grip-** Flat Grip

Technique: Deep Dry Needling

Needle size selection: 0.25mm X 25mm / 0.25mm X 40mm

Needle insertion: The trigger point is palpated for the Interossei muscle and the treatment area is cleaned properly. Needle is tapped into the skin at right angle, Directed towards the muscle belly to elicit a twitch response.

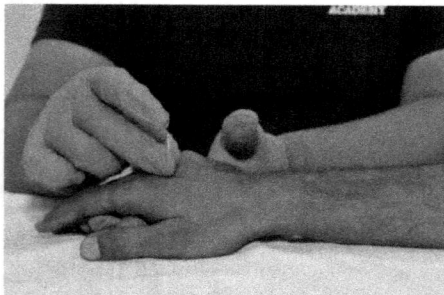

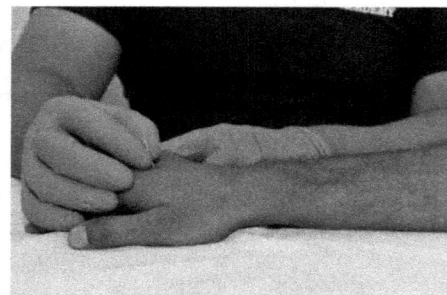

Figure 55: Dry Needling technique of Dorsal Interossei Muscle TrP

CHAPTER 4 - TRIGGER POINT DRY NEEDLING (LOWER QUARTER)

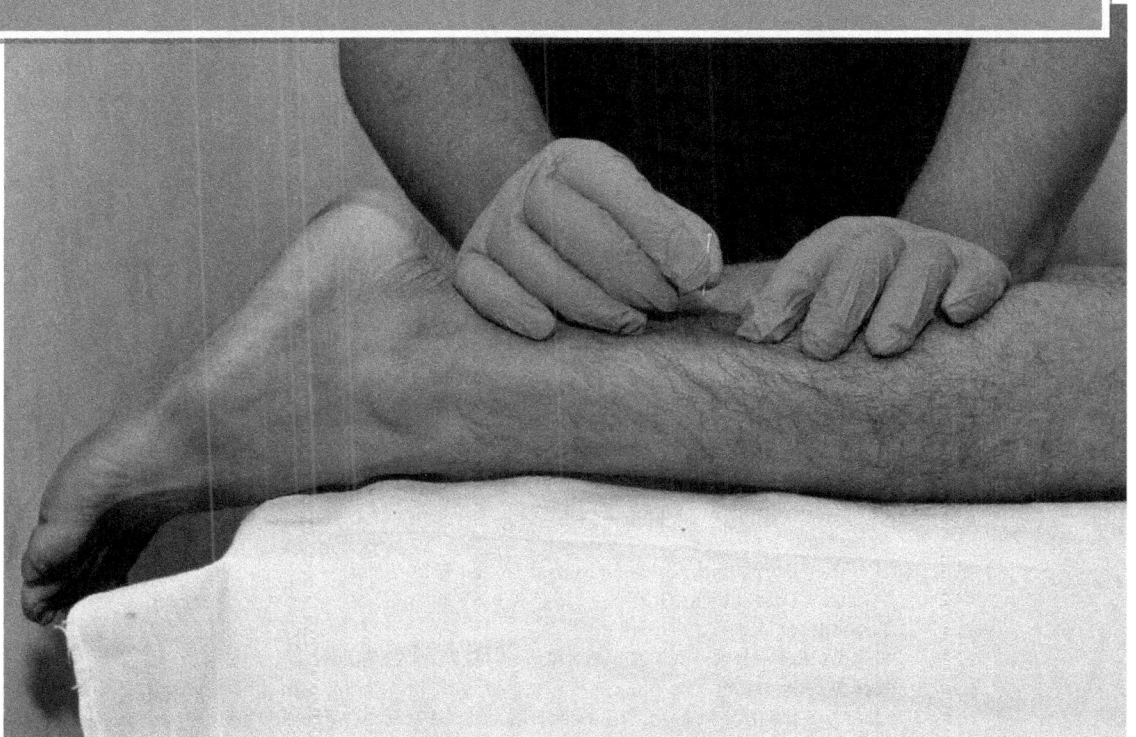

Gluteus Maximus

Basic Anatomy
  Origin:

1. Outer rim of ilium (medial aspect),
2. Dorsal surface of sacrum and coccyx,
3. Sacrotuberous ligament.

Insertion:

1. IT band (primary insertion),
2. Gluteal tuberosity of femur.

Innervations: Inferior gluteal nerve (L5, S1 and S2 nerve roots).
Blood supply: Superior and inferior gluteal arteries.
Function:

1. Powerful extensor & lateral rotator of hip
2. Upper fibers aid in abduction of thigh,
3. Fibers of IT band stabilize a fully extended knee.

Common sites of TrP & Referral pain: Refer to figure 1

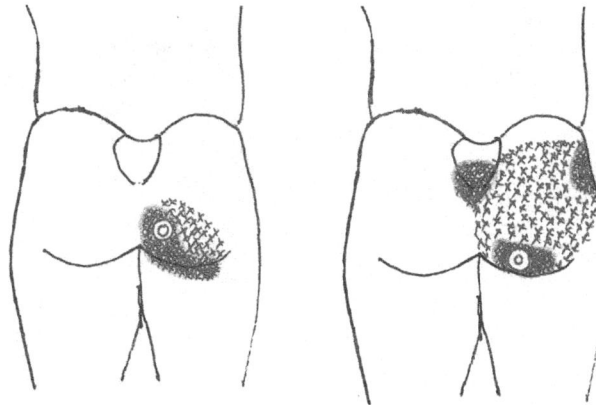

Figure 1: Referral pain of TrP

Procedure
Patient position: Side lying
Palpation:

1. **Bony landmarks-** Sacrum & Ischial Tuburosity
2. **Grip-** Pincer Grip

Technique: Deep Dry Needling
Needle size selection: 0.25mm X 40mm / 0.25mm X 60mm
Needle insertion: The muscle is grasped with one hand with pincer grip and carefully lifted away to clear the treatment area. The needle is tapped at right angle to the belly of muscle. The needle is then manipulated in the muscle belly ensuring it reaches the trigger point to get a localized twitch response.

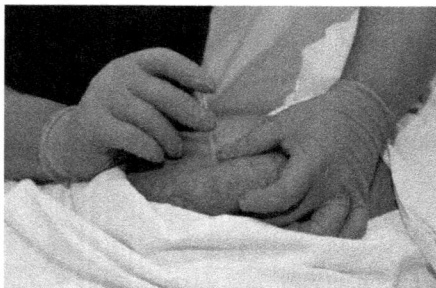

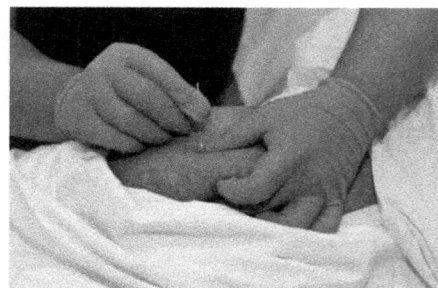

Figure 2: Dry Needling technique of TrP of Gluteus Maximus Muscle

Gluteus Medius

Basic Anatomy

Origin: Outer aspect of ilium (between iliac crest and anterior and posterior gluteal lines),

Insertion: Superior aspect of greater trochanter.

Innervations: Superior gluteal nerve, L4,5, S1.

Blood supply: Superior gluteal artery.

Function:

1. Anterior and lateral fibers abduct and medially rotate the thigh,
2. Stabilizes the pelvis and prevents free limb from sagging during gait.

Common sites of TrP & Referral pain: Refer to figure 3

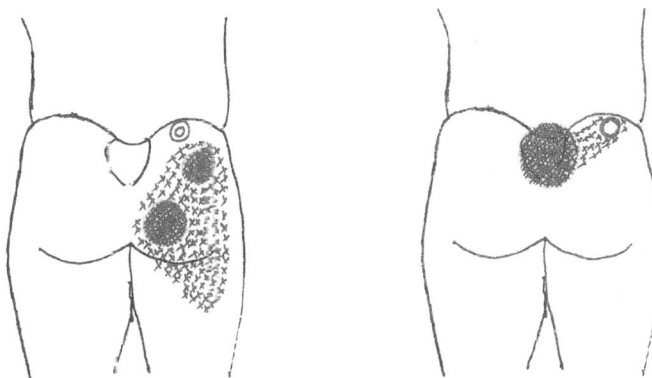

Figure 3: Referral pain of TrP

Procedure

Patient position: Side lying

Palpation:

1. **Bony landmarks-** Sacrum & iliac crest
2. **Grip-** Flat Grip

Technique: Deep Dry Needling

Needle size selection: 0.25mm X 40mm / 0.25mm X 60mm

Needle insertion: The muscle is palpated for trigger point with a flat palpation. The needle is tapped at right angle to the belly of muscle. The needle is directed downwards towards the muscle belly, as it lies beneath gluteus maximus the needle is inserted to cross the muscle, and then it is manipulated in the muscle belly ensuring it reaches the trigger point to get a localized twitch response.

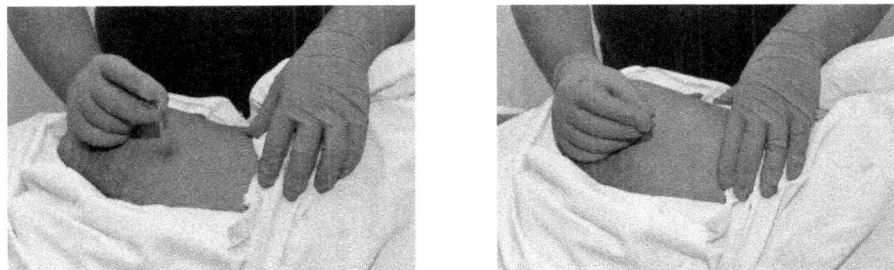

Figure 4: Dry Needling technique of TrP of Gluteus Medius Muscle

Gluteus Minimus

Basic Anatomy

Origin: Outer aspect of ilium (between anterior and inferior gluteal lines).

Insertion:
1. Greater trochanter (anterior to medius),
2. Articular capsule of hip joint.

Innervations: Superior gluteal nerve, L4, 5, S1.

Blood supply: Superior gluteal artery.

Function:
1. Abduct and medially rotate the thigh,
2. Stabilizes the pelvis and prevents free limb from sagging during gait.

Common sites of TrP & Referral pain: Refer to figure 5

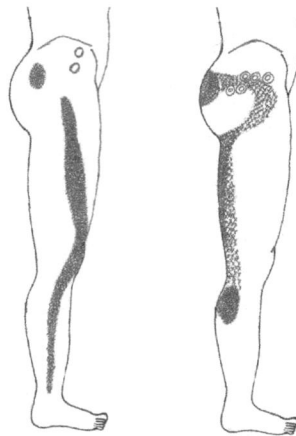

Figure 5: Referral pain of TrP

Procedure

Patient position: Side lying

Palpation:
1. **Bony landmarks-** Sacrum, iliac crest & greater trochanter
2. **Grip-** Flat Grip

Technique: Deep Dry Needling

Needle size selection: 0.25mm X 40mm / 0.25mm X 60mm

Needle insertion: The muscle is palpated for trigger point with a flat palpation. The needle is tapped at right angle to the belly of muscle. The needle is directed directly downwards towards the muscle belly, as it lies beneath gluteus maximus & medius, the needle is inserted to cross the respective muscles, and then it is manipulated in the muscle belly ensuring it reaches the trigger point to get a localized twitch response.

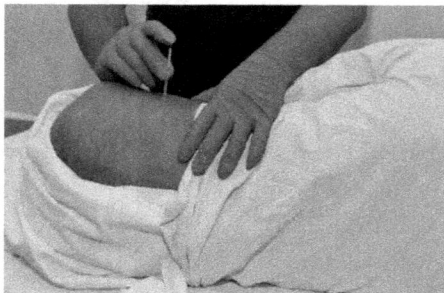

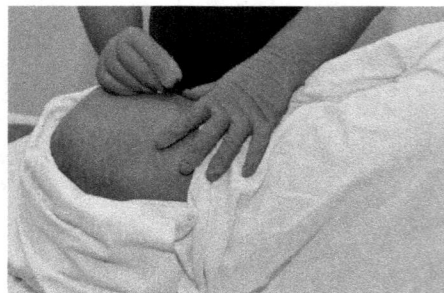

Figure 6: Dry Needling technique of TrP of Gluteus Minimus Muscle

Piriformis

Basic Anatomy

Origin: Pelvic surface of sacrum (anterior portion).

Insertion: Medial surface of greater trochanter (through greater sciatic foramen).

Innervations: Nerve To Piriformis, S1,2.

Blood supply: Inferior gluteal , lateral sacral and superior gluteal artery,

Function:
- Lateral rotation of extended thigh,
- Abducts a flexed thigh.

Common sites of TrP & Referral pain: Refer to figure 7

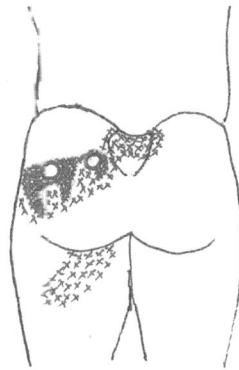

Figure 7: Referral pain of TrP

Procedure

Patient position: Side lying

Palpation:
1. **Bony landmarks-** Sacrum & iliac crest
2. **Grip-** Flat Grip

Technique: Deep Dry Needling

Needle size selection: 0.25mm X 40mm / 0.25mm X 60mm

Needle insertion: The muscle is palpated for trigger point with a flat deep palpation. The needle is tapped at right angle to the belly of muscle. The needle is directed directly downwards towards the muscle belly, as it lies beneath gluteal muscles the needle is inserted to cross the respective muscles, and then it is manipulated in the muscle belly ensuring it reaches the trigger point to get a localized twitch response.

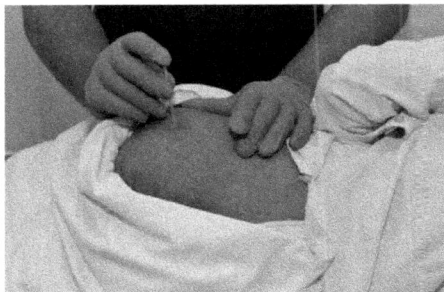

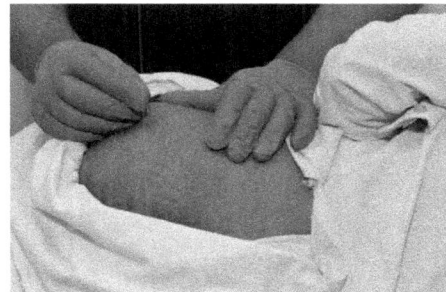

Figure 8: Dry Needling technique of TrP of Piriformis Muscle

Tensor Fascia Lata

Basic Anatomy

Origin: Anterior aspect of iliac crest, ASIS.

Insertion: Anterior aspect of IT band, below greater trochanter.

Innervations: Superior Gluteal Nerve, L4,5,S1.

Blood supply: Primarily lateral circumflex femoral artery, superior gluteal artery.

Function:

1. Hip flexion,
2. Medially rotate & abduct a flexed thigh,
3. Tenses IT tract to support femur on the tibia during standing.

Common sites of TrP & Referral pain: Refer to figure 9

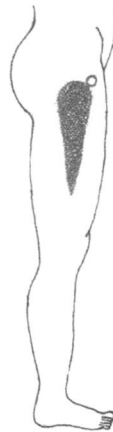

Figure 9: Referral pain of TrP

Procedure

Patient position: Side lying

Palpation:

1. **Bony landmarks-** Iliac crest & greater trochanter
2. **Grip-** Flat Grip

Technique: Deep Dry Needling

Needle size selection: 0.25mm X 40mm / 0.25mm X 60mm

Needle insertion: The muscle is palpated for trigger point with a flat palpation. The needle is tapped at right angle to the belly of muscle. The needle is directed laterally downwards towards the muscle belly then it is manipulated in the muscle belly ensuring it reaches the trigger point to get a localized twitch response.

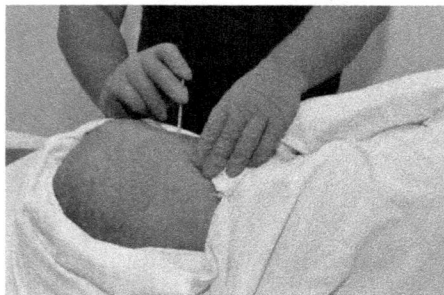

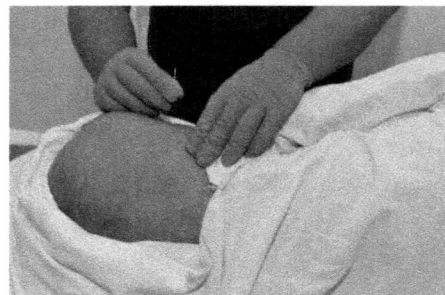

Figure 10: Dry Needling technique of TrP of TFL Muscle

Adductor Magnus

Basic Anatomy
Origin:
1. Pubis symphysis.
2. Tuberosity of the ischium.

Insertion:
1. Linea aspera.
2. Adductor tubercle of femur.

Innervations: Posterior branch of obturator nerve (adductor) and tibial nerve (hamstring).
Blood supply: Deep Femoral Artery.
Function:
1. Adduction of hip (both portions)
2. Flexion of hip (adductor portion)
3. Extension of hip (hamstring portion

Common sites of TrP & Referral pain: Refer to figure 11

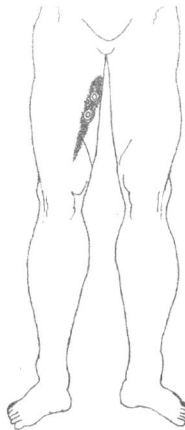

Figure 11: Referral pain of TrP

Procedure
Patient position: Supine lying with hip abducted
Palpation:
1. **Bony landmarks-** Shaft of femur
2. **Grip-** Pincer Grip

Technique: Deep Dry Needling
Needle size selection: 0.25mm X 40mm / 0.25mm X 60mm

Needle insertion: The muscle is palpated for trigger point with a pincer grip. The needle is tapped at right angle to the belly of muscle directed outwards towards the muscle belly then it is manipulated in the muscle belly ensuring it reaches the trigger point to get a localized twitch response.

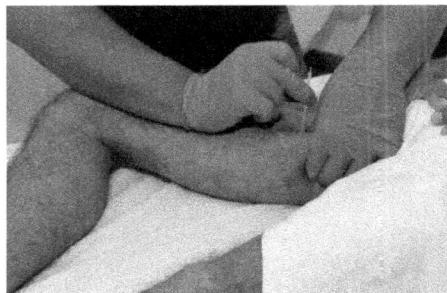

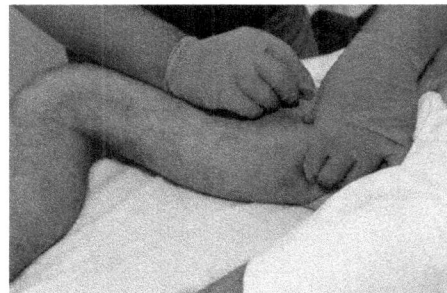

Figure 12: Dry Needling technique of TrP of Adductor Magnus Muscle

Adductor Longus

Basic Anatomy
Origin: Pubic body just below the pubic crest.
Insertion: Middle third of the medial lip of the linea aspera.
Innervations: Anterior branch of obturator nerve.
Blood supply: Deep femoral artery.
Function:
- Adduction of hip,
- Flexion of hip joint.

Common sites of TrP & Referral pain: Refer to figure 13

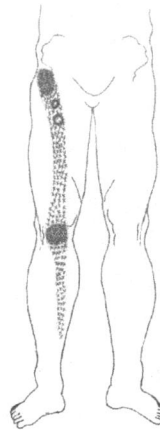

Figure 13: Referral pain of TrP

Procedure
Patient position: Supine lying with hip abducted
Palpation:
1. **Bony landmarks-** Shaft of femur
2. **Grip-** Flat grip

Technique: Deep Dry Needling
Needle size selection: 0.25mm X 40mm / 0.25mm X 60mm

Needle insertion: The muscle is palpated for trigger point with a flat grip. The needle is tapped at right angle to the belly of muscle directed inwards towards the muscle belly then it is manipulated in the muscle belly ensuring it reaches the trigger point to get a localized twitch response.

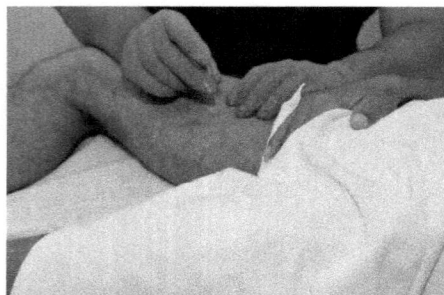

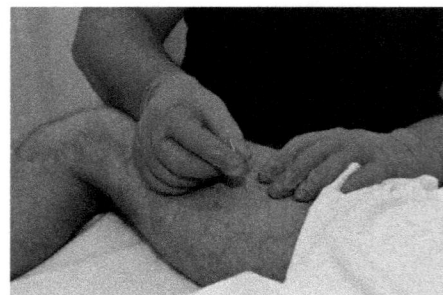

Figure 14: Dry Needling technique of TrP of Adductor Longus Muscle

Pectenius

Basic Anatomy
Origin: Pectineal line of the pubic bone.
Insertion: Pectineal line of the femur.
Innervations: Femoral nerve, sometimes obturator nerve.
Blood supply: Obturator artery
Function: Thigh – Flexion and Adduction.

Common sites of TrP & Referral pain: Refer to figure 15

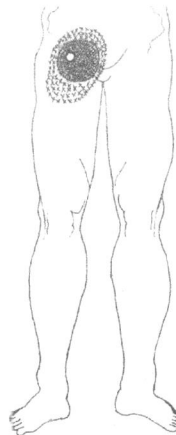

Figure 15: Referral pain of TrP

Procedure
Patient position: Supine Lying with hip abducted
Palpation:
1. **Bony landmarks-** Shaft of femur
2. **Grip-** Flat grip

Technique: Deep Dry Needling
Needle size selection: 0.25mm X 40mm / 0.25mm X 60mm

Needle insertion: The muscle is palpated for trigger point with a flat grip. The needle is tapped at right angle to the belly of muscle directed inwards towards the muscle belly then it is manipulated in the muscle belly ensuring it reaches the trigger point to get a localized twitch response.

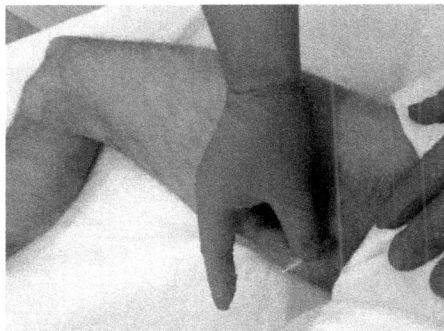

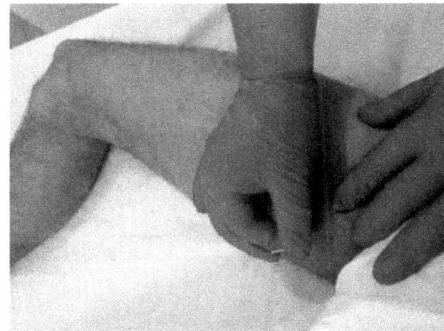

Figure 16: Dry Needling technique of TrP of Pectinius Muscle

Rectus Femoris

Basic Anatomy

Origin: Anterior inferior iliac spine and the exterior surface of the bony ridge which forms the groove on the iliac portion of the acetabulum.

Insertion: Inserts into the patellar tendon as one of the four quadriceps muscles onto tibial tuberosity.

Innervations: Femoral nerve.

Blood supply: Descending branch of the lateral femoral circumflex artery.

Function:
- Knee Extension
- Hip Flexion

Common sites of TrP & Referral pain: Refer to figure 17

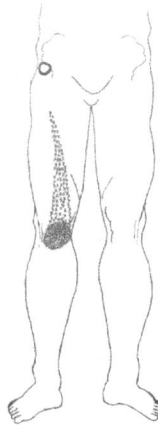

Figure 17: Referral pain of TrP

Procedure

Patient position: Supine Lying

Palpation:
1. **Bony landmarks-** Shaft of femur
2. **Grip-** flat grip

Technique: Deep Dry Needling

Needle size selection: 0.25mm X 40mm / 0.25mm X 60mm

Needle insertion: The muscle is palpated for trigger point with a flat grip. The needle is tapped at right angle to the belly of muscle directed downwards towards the muscle belly then it is manipulated in the muscle belly ensuring it reaches the trigger point to get a localized twitch response.

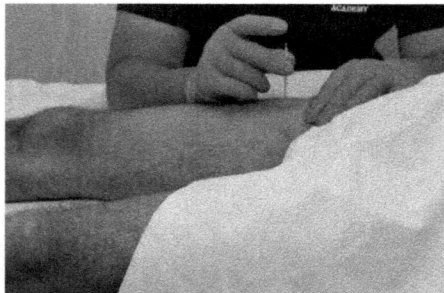

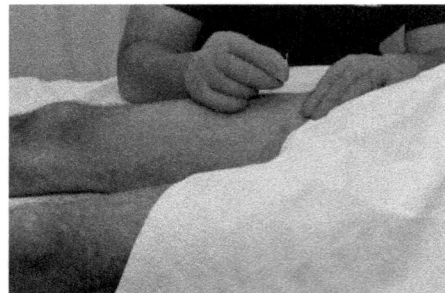

Figure 18: Dry Needling technique of TrP of Rectus Femoris Muscle

Vastus Lateralis

Basic Anatomy

Origin:
1. Greater trochanter,
2. Intertrochanteric line,
3. Linea aspera of the Femur.

Insertion: Patella via the Quadriceps tendon and Tibial tuberosity via the Patellar ligament.

Innervations: Femoral nerve.

Blood supply: Lateral circumflex femoral artery.

Function: Extends and stabilizes knee.

Common sites of TrP & Referral pain: Refer to figure 19

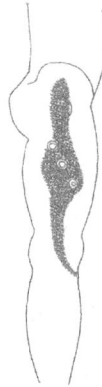

Figure 19: Referral pain of TrP

Procedure

Patient position: Supine Lying

Palpation:
1. **Bony landmarks-** Shaft of femur
2. **Grip-** Pincer grip

Technique: Deep Dry Needling

Needle size selection: 0.25mm X 40mm / 0.25mm X 60mm

Needle insertion: The muscle is palpated for trigger point with a pincer grip. The needle is tapped at right angle to the belly of muscle directed outwards towards the muscle belly then it is manipulated in the muscle belly ensuring it reaches the trigger point to get a localized twitch response.

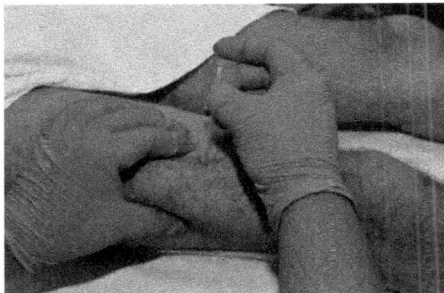

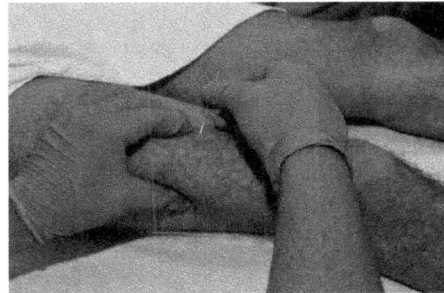

Figure 20: Dry Needling technique of TrP of Vastus Lateralis Muscle

Vastus Medialis

Basic Anatomy

Origin:

1. Lower part of the intertrochanteric line,
2. The spiral line to the medial lip of the linea aspera
3. The medial intermuscular septum
4. The aponeurosis of adductor magnus.

Insertion:

1. Medial side of the quadriceps tendon joining with the rectus femoris and the vasti muscles,
2. The patellar ligament into the tibial tuberosity

Innervations: Femoral nerve.

Blood supply: Femoral artery.

Function: Extension of the leg.

Common sites of TrP & Referral pain: Refer to figure 21

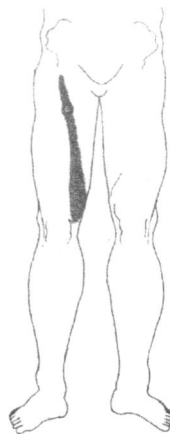

Figure 21: Referral pain of TrP

Procedure

Patient position: Supine Lying

Palpation:

1. **Bony landmarks-** Shaft of femur
2. **Grip-** Pincer grip

Technique: Deep Dry Needling

Needle size selection: 0.25mm X 40mm / 0.25mm X 60mm

Needle insertion: The muscle is palpated for trigger point with a pincer grip. The needle is tapped at right angle to the belly of muscle directed outwards towards the muscle belly then it is manipulated in the muscle belly ensuring it reaches the trigger point to get a localized twitch response.

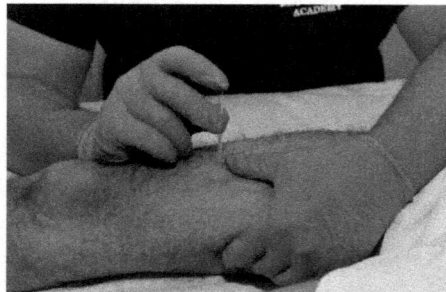

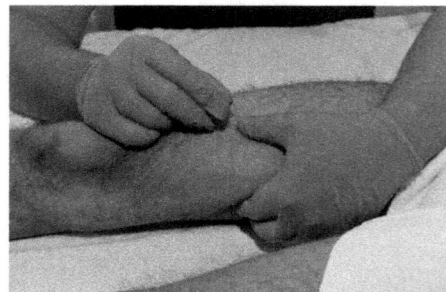

Figure 22: Dry Needling technique of TrP of Vastus Medialis Muscle

Vastus Intermidius

Basic Anatomy

Origin:

1. Anterior and lateral aspects of the upper two-thirds of the femora shaft,
2. The lower part of the lateral intermuscular septum of the femur.

Insertion: Into the quadriceps tendon along with rectus femoris and the other vasti muscles,

Innervations: Femoral nerve.

Blood supply: Femoral artery.

Function: Extension of knee joint.

Common sites of TrP & Referral pain: Refer to figure 23

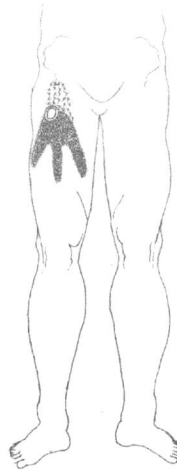

Figure 23: Referral pain of TrP

Procedure

Patient position: Supine Lying

Palpation:

1. **Bony landmarks-** Shaft of femur & patella
2. **Grip-** Flat grip

Technique: Deep Dry Needling

Needle size selection: 0.25mm X 40mm / 0.25mm X 60mm

Needle insertion: The muscle is palpated for trigger point with a flat grip. The needle is tapped at right angle to the belly of muscle directed inwards towards the muscle belly then it is manipulated in the muscle belly ensuring it reaches the trigger point to get a localized twitch response.

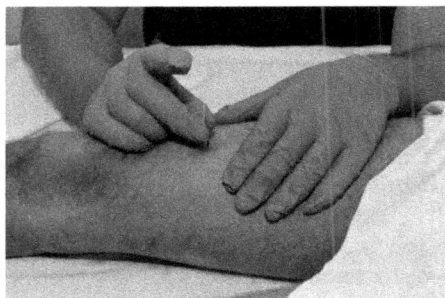

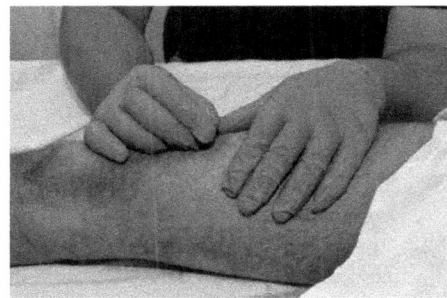

Figure 24: Dry Needling technique of TrP of Vastus Intermedius Muscle

Hamstring

Basic Anatomy

Biceps Femoris:

Origin: Upper and inner surface of the posterior side of the ischial tuberosity, conjoined with semitendinosus.

Insertion: The main attachment is to the styloid process of the fibula, forming a semicircle around the lateral collateral ligament.

Semimembranosus:

Origin: Upper outer quadrant of the posterior surface of the ischial tuberosity,

Insertion: The posterior aspect of the medial condyle of tibia,

Semitensonosus:

Origin: Upper inner quadrant of the posterior surface of the ischial tuberosity,

Insertion: Upper part of the medial surface of the tibia, behind the attachment of the sartorius

Innervations: Tibial nerve, L5,S1,2; Short head of biceps femoris also from common peroneal nerve, L5,S1.

Blood supply: Inferior Gluteal artery, profunda femoris artery.

Common sites of TrP & Referral pain: Refer to figure 25

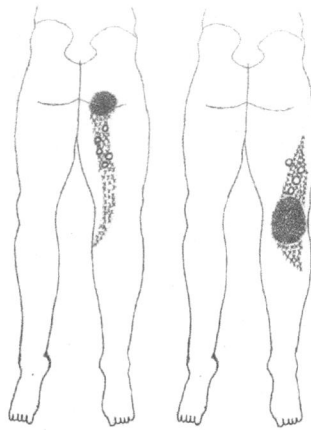

Figure 25: Referral pain of TrP

Procedure

Patient position: Supine Lying

Palpation:

1. **Bony landmarks-** Shaft of femur
2. **Grip-** Pincer grip

Technique: Deep Dry Needling

Needle size selection: 0.25mm X 40mm / 0.25mm X 60mm

Needle insertion:

1. The muscle is palpated for trigger point with a pincer grip. The needle is tapped at right angle to the belly of muscle directed outwards laterally towards the muscle belly then it is manipulated in the muscle belly ensuring it reaches the trigger point to get a localized twitch response. Fig 26
2. The muscle is palpated for trigger point with a pincer grip. The needle is tapped at right angle to the belly of muscle directed outwards medially towards the muscle belly then it is manipulated in the muscle belly ensuring it reaches the trigger point to get a localized twitch response. Fig 27

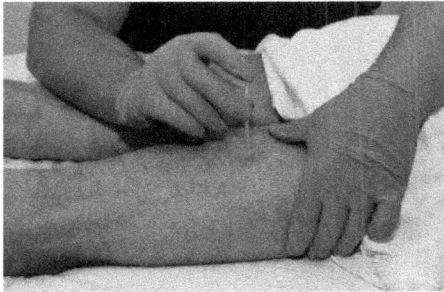

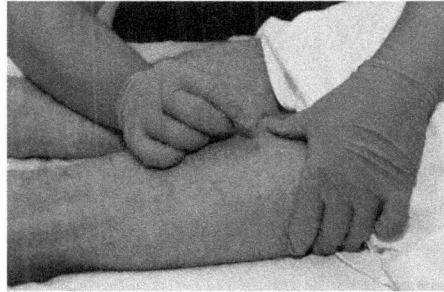

Figure 266: Dry Needling technique of TrP of Biceps Femoris Muscle

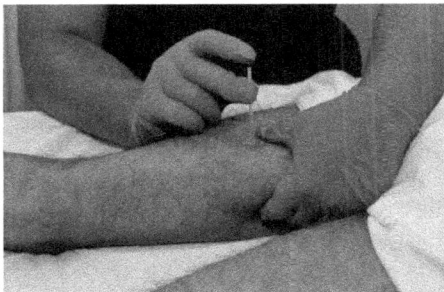

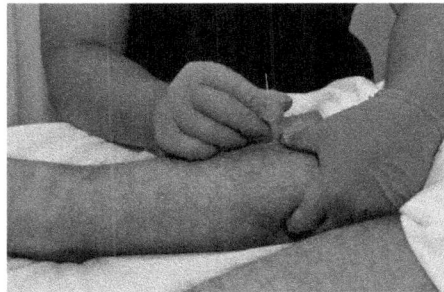

Figure 27: Dry Needling technique of TrP of Semitendinosus & Semimembranus Muscle

Sartorius

Basic Anatomy

Origin: Inferior to the anterior superior iliac spine.

Insertion: Anteromedial surface of the upper tibia in the pes anserinus.

Innervations: Femoral nerve (sometimes from the intermediate cutaneous nerve of thigh).

Blood supply: Femoral artery.

Function:

1. Flexion, abduction, and lateral rotation of the hip,
2. Flexion of the knee.

Common sites of TrP & Referral pain: Refer to figure 28

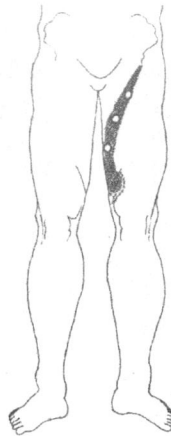

Figure 28: Referral pain of TrP

Procedure

Patient position: Supine Lying

Palpation:

1. **Bony landmarks-** Shaft of femur
2. **Grip-** Flat grip

Technique: Deep Dry Needling

Needle size selection: 0.25mm X 40mm / 0.25mm X 60mm

Needle insertion: The muscle is palpated for trigger point with a flat grip. The needle is tapped at right angle to the belly of muscle directed downwards along the muscle belly, and then it is manipulated in the muscle belly ensuring it reaches the trigger point to get a localized twitch response.

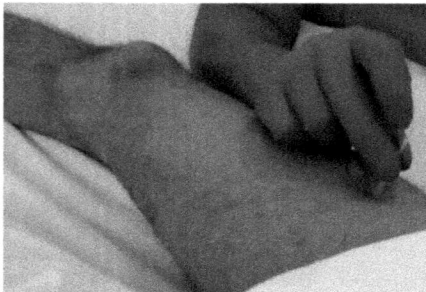

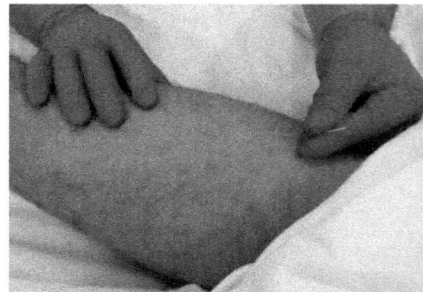

Figure 29: Dry Needling technique of TrP of Sartorius Muscle

Popliteus

Basic Anatomy
Origin:
1. Lateral femoral condyle,
2. Arcuate popliteal ligament,
3. Lateral meniscus,
4. Knee joint capsule.

Insertion: Posterior tibial surface above the soleal line.
Innervations: Tibial nerve, L5, S1.
Blood supply: Popliteal artery.
Function:
1. Insertion fixed: laterally rotates femur on tibia & unlocks knee,
2. Origin fixed: medially rotates tibia on femur & unlocks knee.

Common sites of TrP & Referral pain: Refer to figure 30

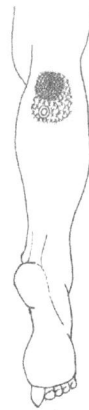

Figure 30: Referral pain of TrP

Procedure
Patient position: Supine Lying with hip abducted & knee flexed
Palpation:
1. **Bony landmarks-** Medial condyle of tibia
2. **Grip-** Flat grip

Technique: Deep Dry Needling
Needle size selection: 0.25mm X 40mm / 0.25mm X 60mm

Needle insertion: The muscle is palpated for trigger point with a flat grip. The needle is tapped and directed inwards towards the muscle belly behind the medial condyle of tibia, and then it is manipulated in the muscle belly ensuring it reaches the trigger point to get a localized twitch response.

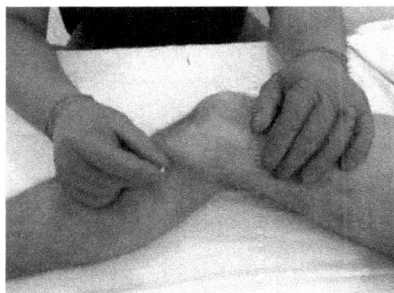

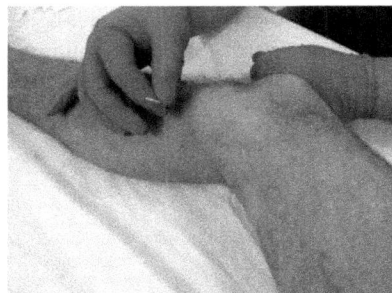

Figure 31: Dry Needling technique of TrP of Popliteus Muscle

Gastrocnemius

Basic Anatomy

Origin:

1. Medial head: just above medial condyle of femur,
2. Lateral head: just above lateral condyle of femur.

Insertion: Calcaneus via lateral portion of calcaneal tendon.

Innervations: Tibial Nerve, S1,2

Blood supply: Sural arteries.

Function:

1. Plantar flex the ankle,
2. Knee flexion (when not weight bearing),
3. Stabilizes ankle & knee when standing.

Common sites of TrP & Referral pain: Refer to figure 32

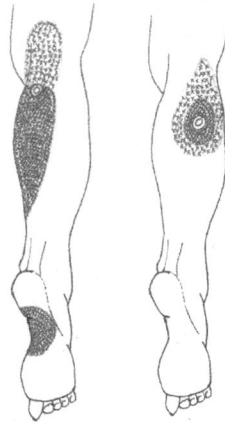

Figure 32: Referral pain of TrP

Procedure

Patient position: Prone Lying

Palpation:

1. **Bony landmarks-** Medial condyle of tibia
2. **Grip-** Pincer grip

Technique: Deep Dry Needling

Needle size selection: 0.25mm X 40mm / 0.25mm X 60mm

Needle insertion:

1. The muscle is palpated for trigger point with a pincer grip. The needle is tapped and directed medially outwards towards the muscle belly, and then it is manipulated in the muscle belly ensuring it reaches the trigger point to get a localized twitch response. The needle should be directed outwards and inwards manipulation should be avoided to prevent injury to tibial nerve & artery. Fig 33

2. The muscle is palpated for trigger point with a pincer grip. The needle is tapped and directed laterally outwards towards the muscle belly, and then it is manipulated in the muscle belly ensuring it reaches the trigger point to get a localized twitch response. The needle should be directed outwards and inwards manipulation should be avoided to prevent injury to tibial nerve & artery. Fig 34

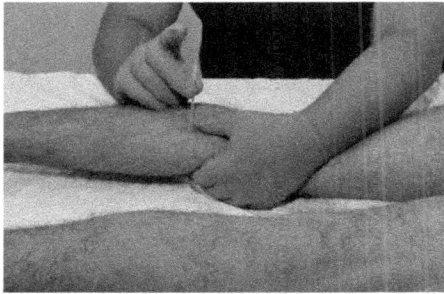

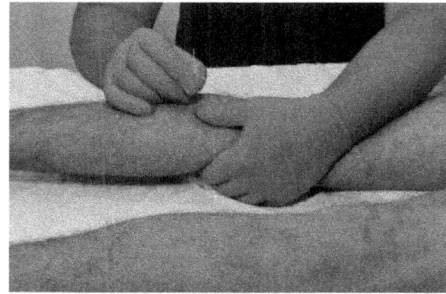

Figure 33: Dry Needing technique of TrP of Gastronemius Muscle (Medial Head)

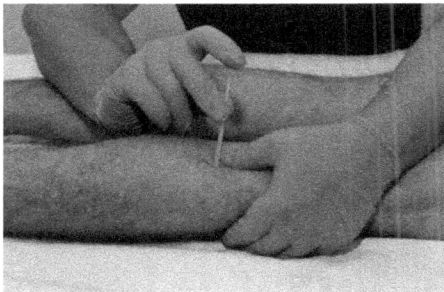

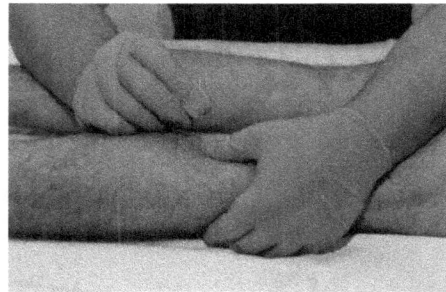

Figure 34: Dry Needling technique of TrP of Gastronemius Muscle (Lateral Head)

Soleus

Basic Anatomy
Origin:
1. Upper fibula,
2. Soleal line of tibia.

Insertion: Calcaneus via medial portion of calcaneal tendon.
Innervations: Tibial Nerve, S1,2.
Blood supply: Sural arteries.
Function: Plantar flex the foot.

Common sites of TrP & Referral pain: Refer to figure 35

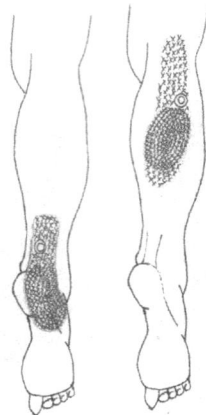

Figure 35: Referral pain of TrP

Procedure
Patient position: Prone Lying
Palpation:
1. **Bony landmarks-** Shaft of Fibula
2. **Grip-** Flat grip

Technique: Deep Dry Needling
Needle size selection: 0.25mm X 40mm / 0.25mm X 60mm

Needle insertion: The muscle is palpated for trigger point with a flat grip. The needle is tapped and directed medially towards the muscle belly just beneath the gastronemius muscle, and then it is manipulated in the muscle belly ensuring it reaches the trigger point to get a localized twitch response. The needle should be directed with precaution to avoid injury to tibial nerve & artery.

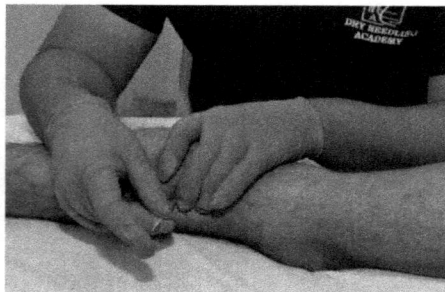

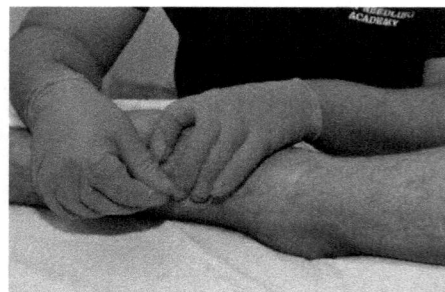

Figure 36: Dry Needling technique of TrP of Soleus Muscle

Plantaris

Basic Anatomy
Origin: Lateral supracondylar ridge of femur above lateral head of gastrocnemius.
Insertion: Tendo calcaneus (medial side, deep to gastrocnemius tendon).
Innervations: Tibial Nerve.
Blood supply: Sural arteries.
Function: Plantar flexes foot and flexes knee.

Common sites of TrP & Referral pain: Refer to figure 37

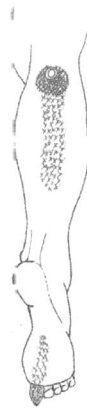

Figure 37: Referral pain of TrP

Procedure
Patient position: Side lying with knee flexed
Palpation:
1. **Bony landmarks-** Tibio-fibular joint
2. **Grip-** Flat grip

Technique: Deep Dry Needling
Needle size selection: 0.25mm X 40mm / 0.25mm X 60mm

Needle insertion: The muscle is palpated for trigger point with a flat grip. The needle is tapped and directed medially towards the muscle belly just below the popliteal fossa, and then it is manipulated in the muscle belly ensuring it reaches the trigger point to get a localized twitch response. The needle should be directed with precaution to avoid injury to tibial nerve & artery.

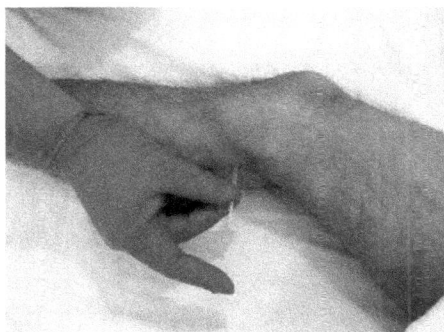

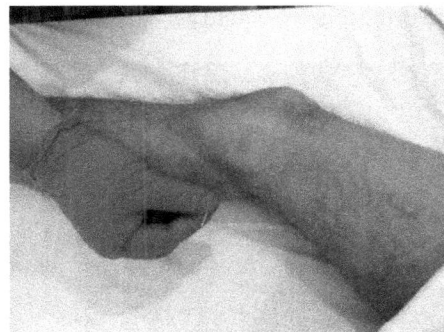

Figure 38: Dry Needling technique of TrP of Plantaris Muscle

Tibialis Anterior

Basic Anatomy

Origin:

1. Lateral condyle and upper half or two-thirds of the lateral surface of the body of the tibia;
2. From the adjoining part of the interosseous membrane;
3. From the deep surface of the fascia;
4. From the intermuscular septum between it and the extensor digitorum longus.

Insertion:

1. Medial and under surface of the medial cuneiform bone,
2. Base of the first metatarsal bone of the foot.

Innervations: Deep Fibular (peroneal) nerve (L4, L5, S1).

Blood supply: Anterior tibial artery.

Function: Dorsiflexion and Inversion of the foot.

Common sites of TrP & Referral pain: Refer to figure 39

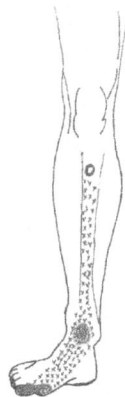

Figure 39: Referral pain of TrP

Procedure

Patient position: Supine lying

Palpation:

1. **Bony landmarks-** shaft of tibia
2. **Grip-** Flat grip

Technique: Deep Dry Needling

Needle size selection: 0.25mm X 25mm / 0.25mm X 40mm

Needle insertion: The muscle is palpated for trigger point with a flat grip. The needle is tapped and directed medially towards the muscle belly, and then it is manipulated in the muscle belly ensuring it reaches the trigger point to get a localized twitch response.

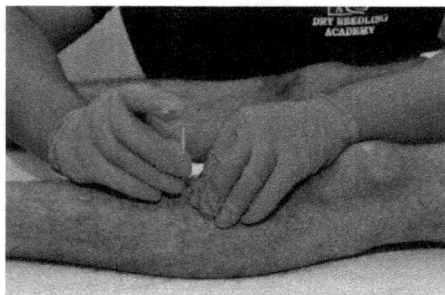

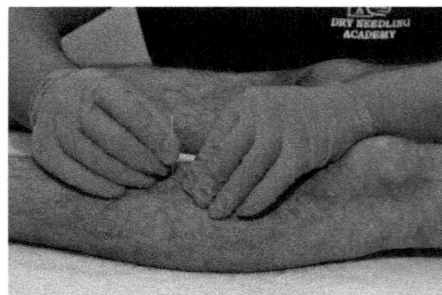

Figure 40: Dry Needling technique of TrP of Tibialis Anterior Muscle

Tibialis Posterior

Basic Anatomy
Origin: On the inner posterior borders of the tibia and fibula.
Insertion: Tuberosity of the navicular and the plantar surface of the first cuneiform.
Innervations: Tibial nerve.
Blood supply: Posterior tibial artery.
Function: Inversion of the foot and plantar flexion of the foot at the ankle.

Common sites of TrP & Referral pain: Refer to figure 41

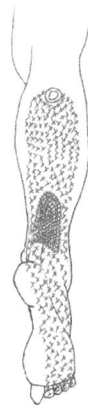

Figure 41: Referral pain of TrP

Procedure
Patient position: Supine lying
Palpation:
1. **Bony landmarks-** shaft of tibia & shaft of fibula
2. **Grip-** Flat grip

Technique: Deep Dry Needling
Needle size selection: 0.25mm X 25mm / 0.25mm X 40mm

Needle insertion: The tibialis posterior is a deep muscle lies beneath the gastronemius and soleus muscle. To needle this muscle an anterior approach is used and the needle is tapped perpendicularly downwards in the tibio-fibular introsseous membrane, then it is directed downwards towards the muscle belly, and then it is manipulated in the muscle belly ensuring it reaches the trigger point to get a localized twitch response.

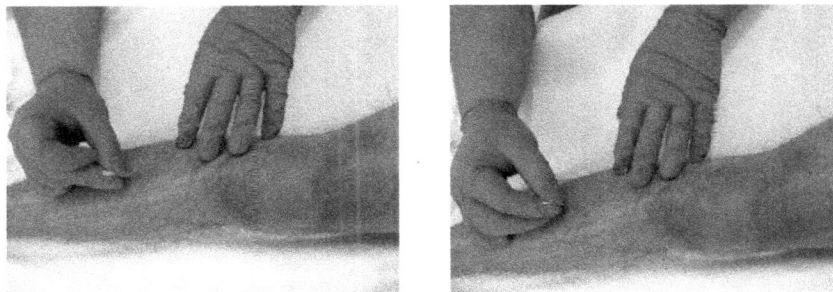

Figure 42: Dry Needling technique of TrP of Tibialis Posterior Muscle

Peroneus Tertius

Basic Anatomy
Origin:
1. Lower third of the anterior surface of the fibula (anterior compartment of lower leg);
2. From the lower part of the interosseous membrane.

Insertion: Base of the fifth metatarsal.
Innervations: Deep peroneal nerve L5, S1.
Blood supply: Anterior tibial artery.
Function: Dorsiflexion and eversion of the foot.

Common sites of TrP & Referral pain: Refer to figure 43

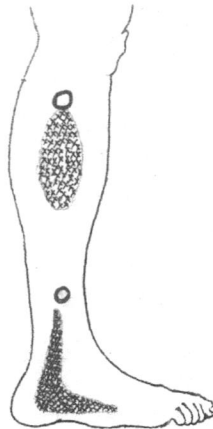

Figure 43: Referral pain of TrP

Procedure
Patient position: Side lying
Palpation:
1. **Bony landmarks-** shaft of fibula
2. **Grip-** Flat grip

Technique: Deep Dry Needling
Needle size selection: 0.25mm X 25mm / 0.25mm X 40mm

Needle insertion: he muscle is palpated for trigger point with a flat grip. The needle is tapped and directed medially towards the muscle belly, and then it is manipulated in the muscle belly ensuring it reaches the trigger point to get a localized twitch response.

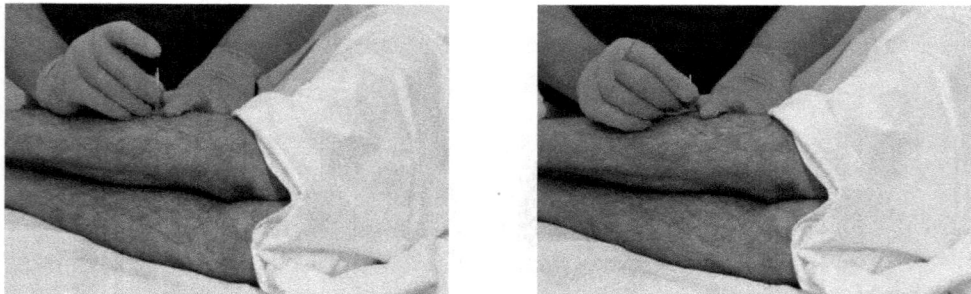

Figure 44: Dry Needling technique of TrP of Peroneus Tertius Muscle

Peroneus Longus

Basic Anatomy

Origin:

- Head and upper two-thirds of the lateral surface of the body of the fibula,
- From the deep surface of the fascia,
- From the intermuscular septa between it and the muscles on the front and back of the leg;
- Upper lateral shaft of fibula.

Insertion: First metatarsal, medial cuneiform.

Innervations: Superficial fibular (peroneal) nerve.

Blood supply: Fibular (peroneal) artery.

Function:

- Plantarflexion,
- Eversion,

Common sites of TrP & Referral pain: Refer to figure 45

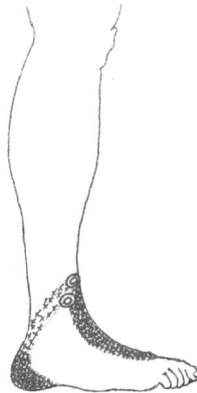

Figure 45: Referral pain of TrP

Procedure

Patient position: Supine lying

Palpation:

1. **Bony landmarks-** shaft of fibula
2. **Grip-** Flat grip

Technique: Deep Dry Needling

Needle size selection: 0.25mm X 25mm / 0.25mm X 40mm

Needle insertion:

The muscle is palpated for trigger point with a flat grip. The needle is tapped and directed downwards towards the muscle belly, and then it is manipulated in the muscle belly ensuring it reaches the trigger point to get a localized twitch response.

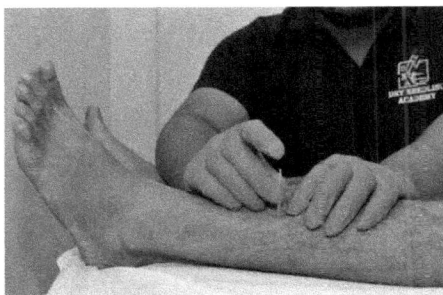

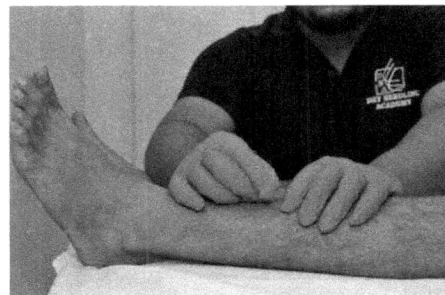

Figure 46: Dry Needling technique of TrP of Peroneus Longus Muscle

Extensor Hallucis Longus

Basic Anatomy
Origin:
- The anterior surface of the fibula for about the middle two-fourths of its extent,
- Medial to the origin of the Extensor digitorum longus;
- Middle portion of the fibula on the anterior surface and the interosseous membrane.

Insertion: Inserts on the dorsal side of the base of the distal phalanx of the big toe.
Innervations: Deep fibular nerve.
Blood supply: Anterior tibial artery.
Function:
- Extends the big toe,
- Assists in dorsiflexion of the foot at the ankle,
- Assists with foot eversion and inversion.

Common sites of TrP & Referral pain: Refer to figure 47

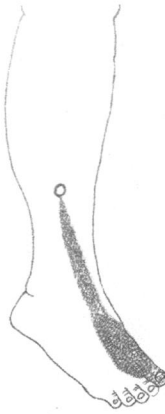

Figure 47: Referral pain of TrP

Procedure
Patient position: Supine lying
Palpation:
1. **Bony landmarks-** shaft of fibula
2. **Grip-** Flat grip

Technique: Deep Dry Needling
Needle size selection: 0.25mm X 25mm / 0.25mm X 40mm

Needle insertion: The muscle is palpated for trigger point with a flat grip. The needle is tapped and directed downwards towards the muscle belly, and then it is manipulated in the muscle belly ensuring it reaches the trigger point to get a localized twitch response.

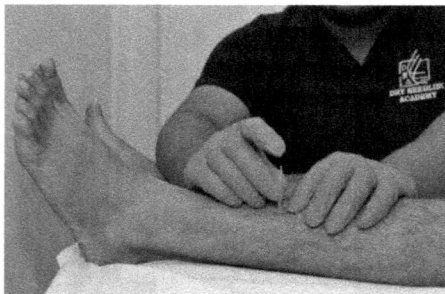

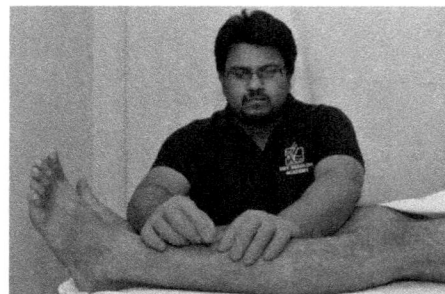

Figure 48: Dry Needling technique of TrP of Extensor Hallucis Longus Muscle

Extensor Digitorum Longus

Basic Anatomy

Origin:

- Anterior lateral condy e of tibia,
- Anterior shaft of fibula and,
- Superior ¾ of interosseous memorane.

Insertion: Dorsal surface; midd e and distal phalanges of lateral four digits.

Innervations: Deep fibular nerve.

Blood supply: Anterior tibial artery.

Function: Extension of toes and dorsiflex on of ankle.

Common sites of TrP & Referral pain: Refer to figure 49

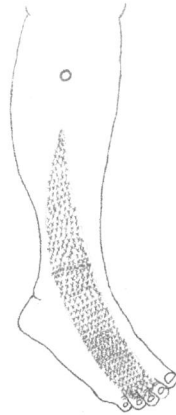

Figure 49: Referral pain of TrP

Procedure

Patient position: Supine lying

Palpation:

1. **Bony landmarks-** Lateral condyle of tibia
2. **Grip-** Flat grip

Technique: Deep Dry Needling

Needle size selection: 0.25mm X 25mm / C.25mm X 40mm

Needle insertion: The muscle is palpated for trigger point with a flat grip. The needle is tapped and directed downwards towards the muscle belly, and then it is manipulated in the muscle belly ensuring it reaches the trigger point to get a localized twitch response.

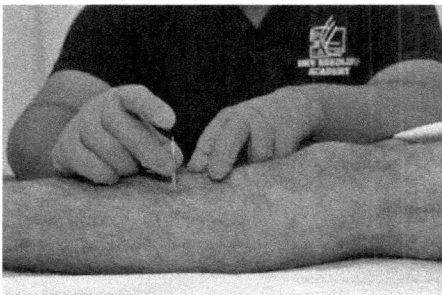

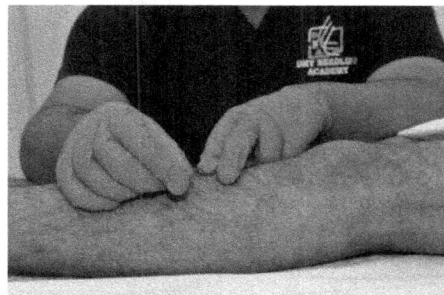

Figure 50: Dry Needling technique of TrP of Extensor Digitorum Longus Muscle

Extensor Digitorum Brevis

Basic Anatomy
Origin: Dorsal surface of calcaneus.
Insertion: Proximal dorsal region of middle phalanges 2, 3 and 4.
Innervations: Deep fibular nerve.
Blood supply: Dorsalis pedis artery.
Function: Extends digits 2 through 4.

Common sites of TrP & Referral pain: Refer to figure 51

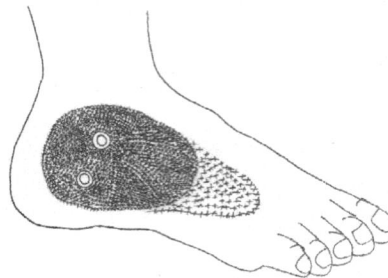

Figure 51: Referral pain of TrP

Procedure
Patient position: Supine lying
Palpation:
1. **Bony landmarks-** lateral malleolus
2. **Grip-** Flat grip

Technique: Deep Dry Needling
Needle size selection: 0.25mm X 25mm

Needle insertion: The muscle is palpated for trigger point with a flat grip. The needle is tapped and directed downwards towards the calcaneum to reach the muscle belly of Extensor digitorum brevis, and then it is manipulated in the muscle belly ensuring it reaches the trigger point to get a localized twitch response.

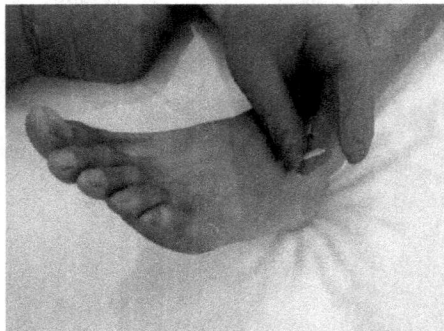

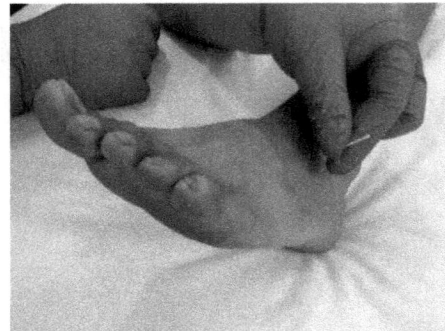

Figure 52: Dry Needling technique of TrP of Extensor Digitorum Brevis Muscle

Flexor Hallucis Longus

Basic Anatomy
Origin: Fibula, posterior aspect of middle 1/3.
Insertion: Plantar surface; base of distal phalanx of hallux.
Innervations: Tibial nerve, S1 & S2 nerve roots.
Blood supply: Peroneal artery ˙peroneal branch of the posterior tibial artery.
Function: Flexes all joints of the big toe, plantar flexion of the ankle joint.

Common sites of TrP & Referral pain: Refer to figure 53

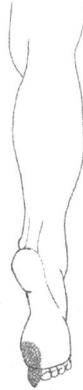

Figure 53: Referral pain of TrP

Procedure
Patient position: Prone lying
Palpation:
1. **Bony landmarks-** lateral malleolus & shaft of fibula
2. **Grip-** Flat grip

Technique: Deep Dry Needling
Needle size selection: 0.25mm X 25mm

Needle insertion: he muscle is palpated for trigger point with a flat grip. The needle is tapped and directed downwards towards the fibula to reach the muscle belly of Flexor hallucis longus, and then it is manipulated in the muscle belly ensuring it reaches the trigger point to get a localized twitch response.

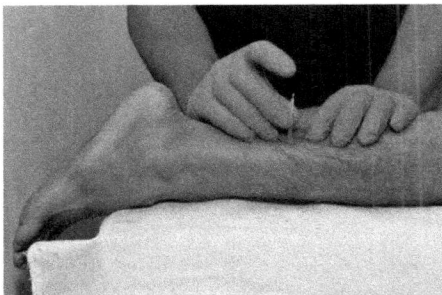

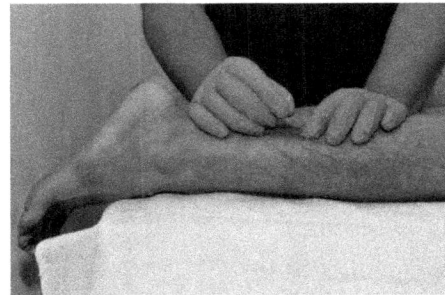

Figure 54: Dry Needling technique of TrP of Flexor Hallucis Longus Muscle

Flexor Hallucis Brevis

Basic Anatomy
Origin:
1. Plantar surface of cuboid
2. Lateral cuneiform bones.

Insertion: Base of proximal phalanx of hallux.
Innervations: Medial plantar nerve.
Blood supply: Medial plantar artery and first plantar metatarsal artery.
Function: Flexion of the metatarsophalangeal joint of the big toe.

Common sites of TrP & Referral pain: Refer to figure 55

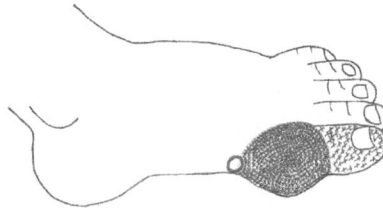

Figure 55: Referral pain of TrP

Procedure
Patient position: side lying
Palpation:
1. **Bony landmarks-** First Metatarsal
2. **Grip-** Flat grip

Technique: Deep Dry Needling
Needle size selection: 0.25mm X 25mm

Needle insertion: The muscle is palpated for trigger point with a flat grip. The needle is tapped and directed downwards towards the Metatarsals to reach the muscle belly of Flexor hallucis brevis, and then it is manipulated in the muscle belly ensuring it reaches the trigger point to get a localized twitch response.

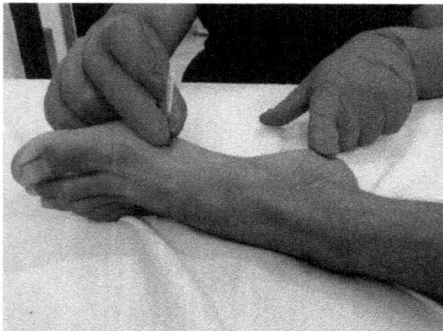

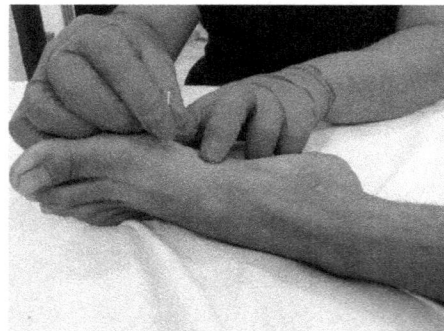

Figure 56: Dry Needling technique of TrP of Flexor Hallucis Brevis Muscle

Extensor Hallucis Brevis

Basic Anatomy
Origin: Dorsal surface of the calcaneus.
Insertion: Dorsal surface of the base of the proximal phalanx of the big toe.
Innervations: Deep peroneal nerve (L5 and S1).
Blood supply:
- The perforating branch of the peroneal artery
- anterior lateral malleolar artery

Function: Assists with extension of the big toe.

Common sites of TrP & Referral pain: Refer to figure 57

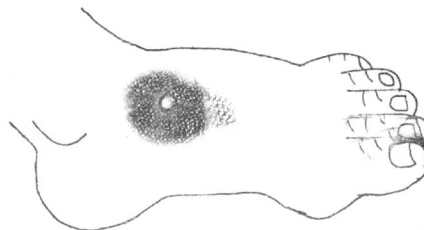

Figure 57: Referral pain of TrP

Procedure
Patient position: Crook Lying/ supine lying
Palpation:
1. **Bony landmarks-** dorsal surface of calcaneum
2. **Grip-** Flat grip

Technique: Deep Dry Needling
Needle size selection: 0.25mm X 25mm

Needle insertion: The muscle is palpated for trigger point with a flat grip. The needle is tapped and directed downwards towards the calcaneum to reach the muscle belly of Extensor hallucis brevis, and then it is manipulated in the muscle belly ensuring it reaches the trigger point to get a localized twitch response.

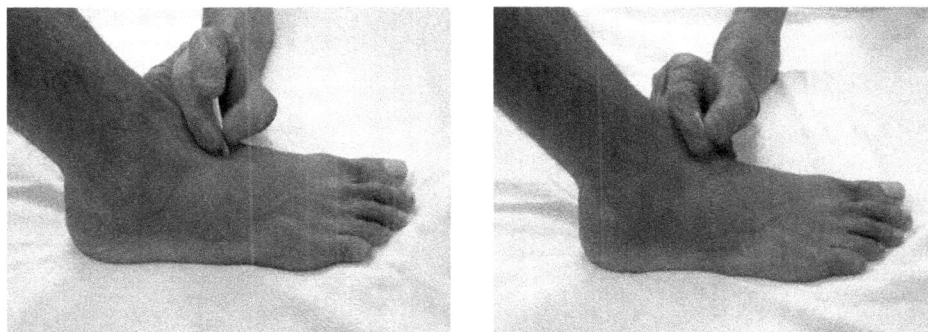

Figure 58: Dry Needling technique of TrP of Extensor Hallucis Brevis Muscle

Adductor Hallucis

Basic Anatomy
Origin:
- Oblique Head: proximal ends of middle 3 metatarsal bones;
- Transverse Head: MTP ligaments of lateral 3 toes.

Insertion: Lateral side of base of first phalanx of the 1st toe.
Innervations: Lateral plantar nerve.
Blood supply: Lateral plantar artery.
Function: Adducts hallux.

Common sites of TrP & Referral pain: Refer to figure 59

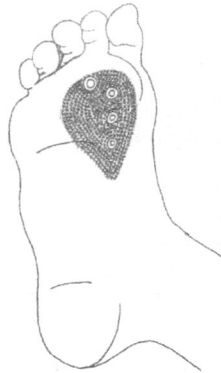

Figure 59: Referral pain of TrP

Procedure
Patient position: Crook Lying/ supine lying
Palpation:
1. **Bony landmarks-** 1st & 2nd Metatarsal
2. **Grip-** Flat grip

Technique: Deep Dry Needling
Needle size selection: 0.25mm X 25mm

Needle insertion: The muscle is palpated for trigger point with a flat grip. The needle is tapped and directed downwards from dorsal to plantar aspect between the 1st & 2nd metatarsal space to reach the muscle belly of Adductor hallucis, and then it is manipulated in the muscle belly ensuring it reaches the trigger point to get a localized twitch response.

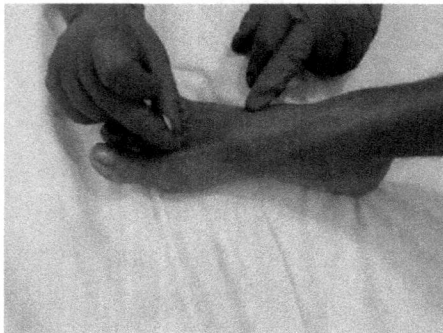

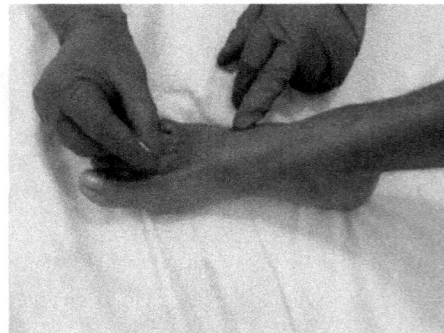

Figure 60: Dry Needling technique of TrP of Adductor Hallucis Muscle

Abductor Hallucis

Basic Anatomy
Origin: Tuberosity of the calcaneus.
Insertion: Medial aspect of base of 1st phalanx of hallux.
Innervations: Medial plantar nerve.
Blood supply: Medial plantar artery.
Function: Abducts hallux.

Common sites of TrP & Referral pain: Refer to figure 61

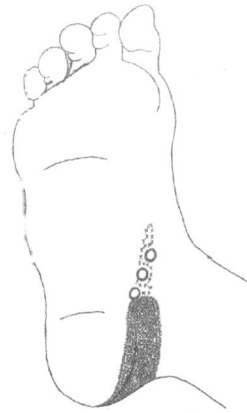

Figure 61: Referral pain of TrP

Procedure
Patient position: Side lying
Palpation:
1. **Bony landmarks-** Medial Side of Calcaneum
2. **Grip-** Flat grip

Technique: Deep Dry Needling
Needle size selection: 0.25mm X 25mm

Needle insertion: The muscle is palpated for trigger point with a flat grip. The needle is tapped and directed downwards towards the medial surface of first metatarsal to reach the muscle belly of Abductor hallucis, and then it is manipulated in the muscle belly ensuring it reaches the trigger point to get a localized twitch response.

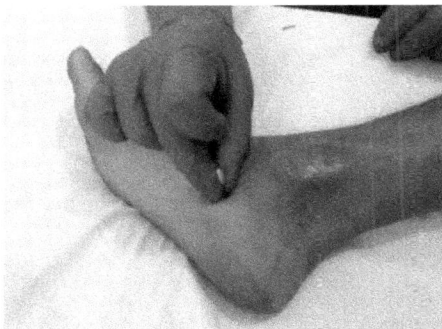

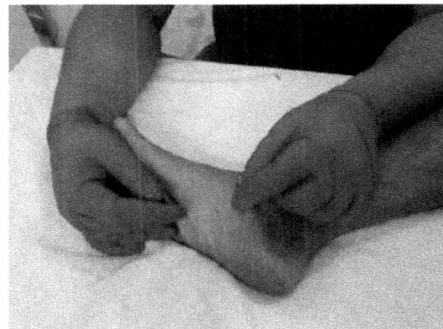

Figure 62: Dry Needling technique of TrP of Abductor Hallucis Muscle

Flexor Digitorum Brevis

Basic Anatomy
Origin:
1. Medial aspect of calcaneal tuberosity
2. The deep surface of the plantar aponeurosis.

Insertion: Attaches to the middle phalanx.
Innervations: Medial plantar nerve (S1 and S2).
Blood supply:
- The belly of the muscle receives blood from the lateral and medial plantar arteries and the plantar metatarsal arteries.
- The tendons are supplied by the plantar digital arteries.

Function: Flexion of metatarsophalangeal joints and proximal interphalangeal joints of toes 2, 3, & 4

Common sites of TrP & Referral pain: Refer to figure 63

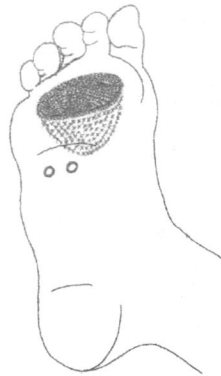

Figure 63: Referral pain of TrP

Procedure
Patient position: Side lying
Palpation:
1. **Bony landmarks-** 2nd, 3rd & 4th Metatarsal
2. **Grip-** Flat grip

Technique: Deep Dry Needling
Needle size selection: 0.25mm X 25mm

Needle insertion: The muscle is palpated for trigger point with a flat grip. The needle is tapped and directed from plantar to dorsal aspect between the 3rd & 4th metatarsal space to reach the muscle belly of Flexor digitorum brevis, and then it is manipulated in the muscle belly ensuring it reaches the trigger point to get a localized twitch response.

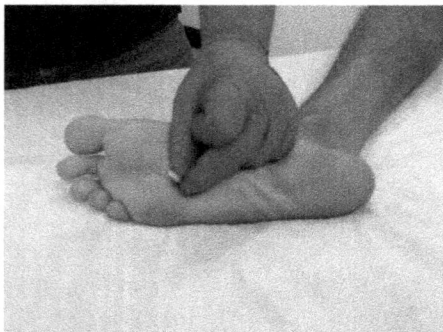

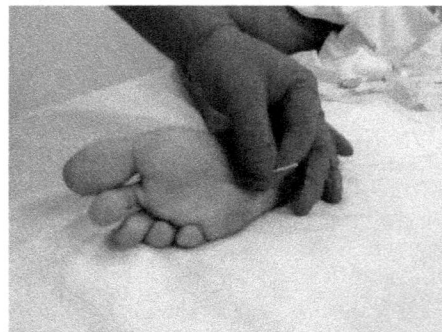

Figure 64: Dry Needling technique of TrP of Flexor Digitorum Brevis Muscle

Abductor Digiti Minimi

Basic Anatomy
Origin: Plantar aponeurosis.
Insertion: Fifth toe or phalanges.
Innervations: Lateral plantar nerve.
Blood supply: Lateral plantar artery.
Function: Flexion and abduction of the fifth toe.

Common sites of TrP & Referral pain: Refer to figure 65

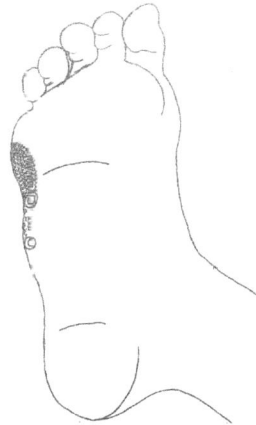

Figure 65: Referral pain of TrP

Procedure
Patient position: Side lying
Palpation:
1. **Bony landmarks-** Lateral surface of calcaneum
2. **Grip-** Flat grip

Technique: Deep Dry Needling
Needle size selection: 0.25mm X 25mm

Needle insertion: The muscle is palpated for trigger point with a flat grip. The needle is tapped and directed downwards from lateral aspect to reach the muscle belly of Abductor digiti minimi, and then it is manipulated in the muscle belly ensuring it reaches the trigger point to get a localized twitch response.

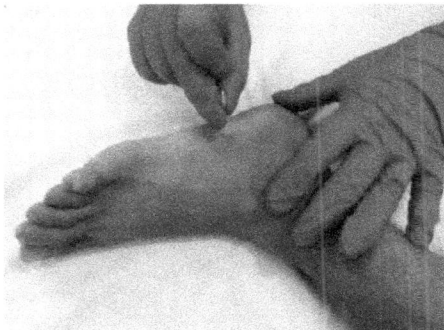

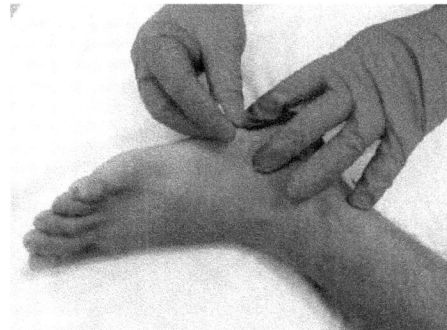

Figure 66: Dry Needling technique of TrP of Abductor Digiti Minimi Muscle

Quadratus Plantae

Basic Anatomy
Origin:
1. Lateral head-tuberosity of calcaneus,
2. Medial head-medial side of calcaneus

Insertion: Lateral border long flexor tendons
Innervations: Lateral plantar (S2,S3)
Blood supply: Lateral plantar artery.
Function: Flexion of toes.

Common sites of TrP & Referral pain: Refer to figure 67

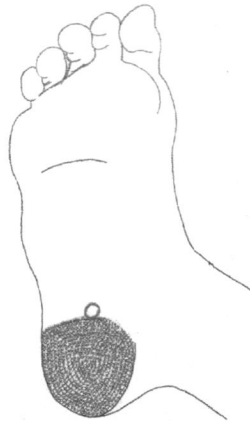

Figure 67: Referral pain of TrP

Procedure
Patient position: supine lying
Palpation:
1. **Bony landmarks-** dorsal surface of calcaneum
2. **Grip-** Flat grip

Technique: Deep Dry Needling
Needle size selection: 0.25mm X 25mm

Needle insertion: The muscle is palpated for trigger point with a flat grip. The needle is tapped and directed from planter aspect to reach the muscle belly of Quadratus plantae, and then it is manipulated in the muscle belly ensuring it reaches the trigger point to get a localized twitch response.

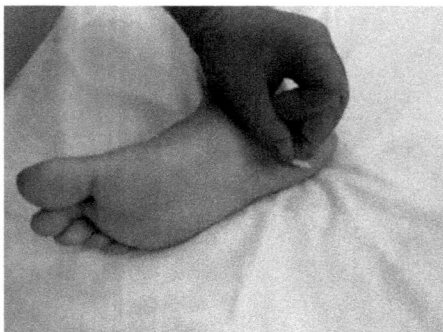

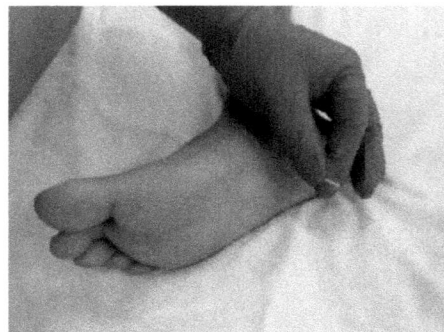

Figure 68: Dry Needling technique of TrP of Quadratus Plantae Muscle

Dorsal & Plantar Interossei

Basic Anatomy
Dorsal Interossei
Origin: Two heads from the proximal ha f of the sides of adjacent metatarsal bones
Insertion: The bases of the second, thir⸱, and fourth proximal phalanges
Innervations: Lateral plantar nerve (S2,S3)
Blood supply: Lateral plantar artery.
Function: Abduct 2nd, 3rd and 4th toes from axis of 2nd toe. Assist lumbricals in extending interphalangeal joints while flexing metatarsal phalangeal joints

Plantar Interossei
Origin: Inferomedial shafts of 3rd, 4th and 5th metatarsals
Insertion: Medial sides of bases of proximal phalanges with slips to dorsal extensor expansions of 3rd, 4th and 5th toes
Innervations: Lateral plantar nerve (S2,S3)
Blood supply: Lateral plantar artery.
Function: Adduct 3rd 4th and 5th toes to axis of 2nd toe, Assist lumbricals in extending interphalangeal joints while flexing metatarsal phalangeal joints

Common sites of TrP & Referral pain: Refer to figure 69

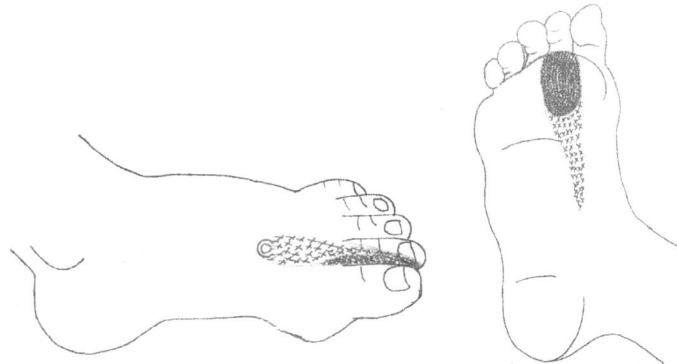

Figure 69: Referral pain of TrP

Procedure
Patient position: Supine lying / Side Lying
Palpation:
1. **Bony landmarks-** Metatarsals
2. **Grip-** Flat grip
Technique: Deep Dry Needling
Needle size selection: 0.25mm X 25mm

Needle insertion:
1. The muscle is palpated for trigger point with a flat grip. The needle is tapped and directed downwards from dorsal aspect to reach the muscle belly of dorsal interossei, and then it is manipulated in the muscle belly ensuring it reaches the trigger point to get a localized twitch response. Fig 70
2. The muscle is palpated for trigger point with a flat grip. The needle is tapped and directed upwards from plantar aspect to reach the muscle belly of plantar interossei, and then it is manipulated in the muscle belly ensuring it reaches the trigger point to get a localized twitch response. Fig 71

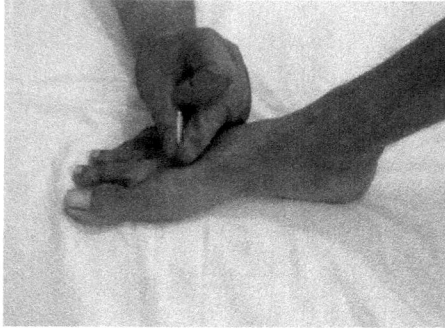

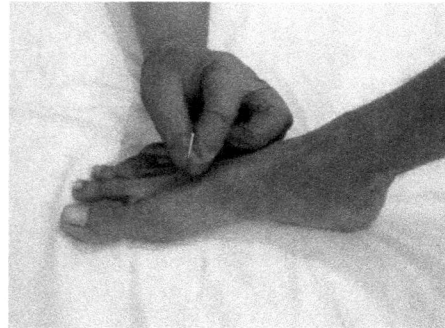

Figure 70: Dry Needling technique of TrP of Dorsal interossei Muscle

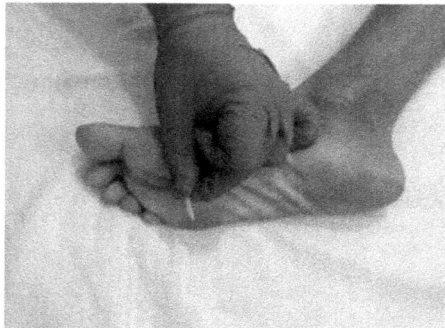

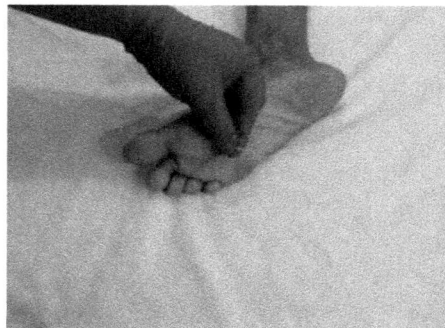

Figure 71: Dry Needling technique of TrP of Plantar interossei Muscle

SUGGESTIVE READING

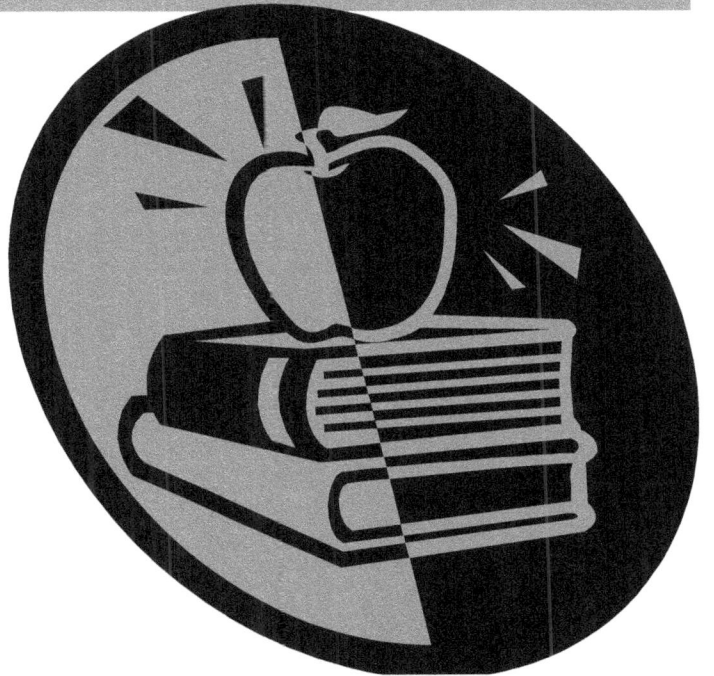

Suggestive Reading

1. A. Feldreich, M. Ernberg, B. Lund, and A. Rosen, "Increased beta-endorphin levels and generalized decreased pain thresholds in patients with limited jaw opening and movement-evoked pain from the temporomandibular joint," Journal of Oral and Maxillofacial Surgery, vol. 70, no. 3, pp. 547–556, 2012.

2. A. Inoue, K. Ikoma, N. Morioka et al., "Interleukin-1β induces substance P release from primary afferent neurons through the cyclooxygenase-2 system," Journal of Neurochemistry, vol. 73, no. 5, pp. 2206–2213, 1999.

3. A. Krebs andW. A. Johnson, "Metabolism of ketonic acids in animal tissues," The Biochemical Journal, vol. 31, no. 4, pp. 645–660, 1937.

4. A. Malanga and E. J. C. Colon, "Myofascial low back pain: a review," Physical Medicine and Rehabilitation Clinics of North America, vol. 21, no. 4, pp. 711–724, 2010.

5. A. S. McMillan, A. Nolan, and P. J. Kelly, "The efficacy of dry needling and procaine in the treatment of myofascial pain in the jaw muscles," Journal of Orofacial Pain, vol. 11, no. 4, pp. 307–314, 1997.

6. A. Sluka, A. Kalra, and S. A. Moore, "Unilateral intramuscular injections of acidic saline produce a bilateral, long-lasting hyperalgesia," Muscle & Nerve, vol. 24, no. 1, pp. 37–46, 2001.

7. A. Sluka, M. P. Price, N. M. Breese, C. L. Stucky, J. A. Wemmie, and M. J. Welsh, "Chronic hyperalgesia induced by repeated acid injections in muscle is abolished by the loss of ASIC3, but not ASIC1," Pain, vol. 106, no. 3, pp. 229–239, 2003.

8. A. Stofan, L. A. Callahan, A. F. DiMarco, D. E. Nethery, and G. S. Supinski, "Modulation of release of reactive oxygen species by the contracting diaphragm," American Journal of Respiratory and Critical Care Medicine, vol. 161, no. 3, part 1, pp. 891–898, 2000.

9. Adair-Kirk TL, Senior RM. Fragments of extracellular matrix as mediators of inflammation. Int J Biochem Cell Biol. 2008;40(6-7):1101-1110.

10. Affaitati G, Costantini R, Fabrizio A, Lapenna D, Tafuri E, Giamberardino MA. Effects of treatment of peripheral pain generators in fibromyalgia patients. Eur J Pain. Jan 2011;15(1):61-69.

11. Akki, M. Zhang, C. Murdoch, A. Brewer, and A. M. Shah, "NADPH oxidase signaling and cardiac myocyte function," Journal of Molecular and Cellular Cardiology, vol. 47, no. 1, pp. 15–22, 2009.

12. Alberts and S. O. ¨ Ogren, "Effects of alaproclate, potassium channel blockers, and lidocaine on the release of 3Hacetylcholine from the guinea-pig ileum myenteric plexus," Pharmacology & Toxicology, vol. 65, no. 1, pp. 25–32, 1989.

13. Alijevic and S. Kellenberger, "Subtype-specific modulation of acid-sensing ion channel (ASIC) function by 2-guanidine-4-methylquinazoline," The Journal of Biological Chemistry, vol. 287, no. 43, pp. 36059–36070, 2012.

14. Andersen SA. Bilateral pneumothorax associated to acupuncture. Ugeskr Laeger. 2011;173(43):2724–5.

15. Ay S, Evcik D, Tur BS. Comparison of injection methods in myofascial pain syndrome: a randomized controlled trial. Clin Rheumatol. 2010;29(1):19–23.

16. Bajaj P, Bajaj P, Graven-Nielsen T, Arendt-Nielsen L. Trigger points in patients with lower limb osteoarthritis. J Musculoskeletal Pain. 2001;9(3):17-33.

17. Baldry PE. Acupuncture, Trigger Points and Musculoskeletal Pain. Edinburgh: Churchill Livingstone; 2005.

18. Ballyns JJ, Shah JP, Hammond J, Gebreab T, Gerber LH, Sikdar S. Objective sonographic measures for characterizing myofascial trigger points associated with cervical pain. J Ultrasound Med. Oct 2011;30(10):1331-1340.

19. Ballyns JJ, Turo D, Otto P, et al. Office-based elastographic technique for quantifying mechanical properties of skeletal muscle. J. Ultrasound Med. Aug 2012;31(8):1209-1219.

20. Baron, "Mechanisms of disease: neuropathic pain—a clinical perspective," Nature Clinical Practice Neurology, vol. 2, no. 2, pp. 95–106, 2006.

21. Baron, "Peripheral neuropathic pain: from mechanisms to symptoms," Clinical Journal of Pain, vol. 16, no. 2, pp. S12–S20, 2000.

22. Bayeva and H. Ardehali, "Mitochondrial dysfunction and oxidative damage to sarcomeric proteins," CurrentHypertens on Reports, vol. 12, no. 6, pp. 426–432, 2010.

23. Bear MF, Connors BW, Paraciso MA. Neuroscience: Exploring the Brain. 3rd ed. Philadelphia: Lippincott Williams & Wilkins, 2007.

24. Betts D, Budd S. 'Forbidden points' in pregnancy: historical wisdom? Acupunct Med. 2011; 29:137-139.

25. Bjorkedal E, Flaten MA. Expectations of increased and decreased pain explain the effect of conditioned pain modulation in females. J Pain Res. 2012;5:289-300.

26. Blumenfeld H. Neuroanatomy through Clinical Cases. Massachusetts: Sinauer Associates. Inc., 2002.

27. Borg-Stein and D. G. Simons, "Focused review: myofascial pain," Archives of Physical Medicine and Rehabilitation, vol. 83, supplement 1, no. 3, pp. S40–S47, 2002.

28. Brady, S., McEvoy, J., Dommerholt, J., Doody, C.: Adverse events following trigger point dry needling: a prospective survey of chartered physiotherapists. submitted, 2012

29. Brückle W, Sückfull M, Fleckenstein W, Weiss C, Müller W. Gewebe-pO2-Messung in der verspannten Rückenmuskulatur (m. erector spinae). Z. Rheumatol. 1990;49:208-216.

30. Bukharaeva EA, Salakhutdinov RI, Vyskocil F, Nikolsky EE. Spontaneous quantal and non-quantal release of acetylcholine at mouse endplate during onset of hypoxia. Physiol Res. 2005;54(2):251- 255.

31. C. Gomez-Cabrera, G. L. Close, A. Kayani, A. McArdle, J. Vi~na, and M. J. Jackson, "Effect of xanthine oxidase-generated extracellular superoxide on skeletal muscle force generation," American Journal of Physiology: Regulatory Integrative and Comparative Physiology, vol. 298, no. 1, pp. R2–R8, 2010.

32. C. Poole, T. I. Musch, and C. A. Kindig, "In vivo microvascular structural and functional consequences of muscle length changes," The American Journal of Physiology—Heart and Circulatory Physiology. vol. 272, no. 5, pp. H2107–H2114, 1997.

33. C. Z. Hong and Y. Torizoe, "Electrophysiological characteristics of localized twitch responses in responsive taut bands of rabbit skeletal muscle fibers," Journal of Musculoskeletal Pain, vol. 2, no. 2, pp. 17–43, 1994.

34. C. Z. Hong, "Lidocaine injection versus dry needling to myofascial trigger point: the importance of the local twitch response," American Journal of Physical Medicine and Rehabilitation, vol. 73, no. 4, pp. 256–263, 1994.

35. C. Z. Hong, "New trends in myofascial pain syndrome," Chinese Medical Journal, vol. 65, no. 11, pp. 501–512, 2002.

36. C. Couppe, A. Midttun, J.Hilden, U. Jørgensen, P. Oxholm, and A. Fuglsang-Frederiksen, "Spontaneous needle electromyographic activity inmyofascial trigger points in the infraspinatus muscle: a blinded assessment," Journal of Musculoskeletal Pain, vol. 9, no. 3, pp. 7–16, 2001.

37. Calandre EP, Hidalgo J. Garcia-Leiva JM, Rico-Villademoros F. Trigger point evaluation in migraine patients: an indication of peripheral sensitization linked to migraine predisposition?Eur J Neurol. Mar 2006;13(3):244-249.

38. Capuano, D. Curr'o, C. Dello Russo et al., "Nociceptin (1–13)NH2 inhibits stimulated calcitonin-gene- related-peptide release from primary cultures of rat trigeminal ganglia neurones," Cephalalgia, vol. 27, no. 8, pp. 868–876, 2007.

39. Ceccherelli F, Rigoni MT. Gagliardi G, Ruzzante L. Comparison between superficial and deep acupuncture in the treatment of lumbar myofascial pain: a double-blind randomized controlled study. Clin J Pain. 2002;18:149-153.

40. Celik and E. K. Mutlu, "Clinical implication of latent myofascial trigger point," Current Pain and Headache Reports, vol. 17, no 8, article 353, 2013.

41. Chan MW, Hinz B, McCulloch CA. Mechanical induction of gene expression in connective tissue cells. Methods Cell Biol. 2010;98:178-205.

42. Chen JT, Chung KC, Hou CR, Kuan TS, Chen SM, Hong CZ. Inhibitory effect of dry needling on the spontaneous electrical activity recorded from myofascial trigger spots of rabbit skeletal muscle. Am J Phys Med Rehabil. Oct 2001;80(10):729-735.

43. Chen Q, Basford J, An KN. Ability of magnetic resonance elastography to assess taut bands. Clin Biomech (Bristol, Avon). 2008;23(5):623-629.

44. Chen Q, Bensamoun S, Basford JR, Thompson JM, An KN. Identification and quantification of myofascial taut bands with magnetic resonance elastography. Arch Phys Med Rehabil. 2007;88(12):1658–61.

45. Chen SM, Chen JT, Kuan TS, Hong CZ. Myofascial trigger points in intercostal muscles secondary to herpes zoster infection of the intercostal nerve. Arch Phys Med Rehabil. 1998;79(3):336-338.

46. Chiquet M, Renedo AS, Huber F, Fluck M. How do fibroblasts translate mechanical signals into changes in extracellular matrix production? Matrix Biol. Mar 2003;22(1):73-80.

47. Cicerone KD. Evidence-based practice and the limits of rational rehabilitation. Arch Phys Med Rehabil. Jun 2005;86(6):1073-1074.

48. Cummings M. 'Forbidden points' in pregnancy: no plausible mechanism for risk. Acupunct Med.2011;29:140-142.

49. Cummings TM, White AR. Needling therapies in the management of myofascial trigger point pain: a systematic review. Arch Phys Med Rehabil. 2001;82(7):986–92.

50. D. Bullock, "Relative afferent pupillary defect in the "better" eye," Journal of Clinical Neuro-Ophthalmology, vol. 10, no. 1, pp. 45–51, 1990.

51. D. Crane, D. I. Ogborn, C. Cupido et al., "Massage therapy attenuates inflammatory signaling after exercise-induced muscle damage.," Science Translational Medicine, vol. 4, no. 119, pp.119–ra13, 2012. 14 International Scholarly Research Notices

52. D. G . Simons, J. G. Travell, L. S. Simons, and B. D. Cummings, Travell & Simons' Myofascial Pain and Dysfunction:The Trigger Point Manual, LippincottWilliams &Wilkins, 1998.

53. D. G. Simons and W. C. Stolov, "Microscopic features and transient contraction of palpable bands in canine muscle," American Journal of Physical Medicine, vol. 55, no. 2, pp. 65–88, 1976.

54. D. G. Simons, "Clinical and etiological update of myofascial pain from trigger points," Journal of Musculoskeletal Pain, vol. 4, no. 1-2, pp. 93–121, 1996.

55. D. G. Simons, "Review of enigmaticMTrPs as a common cause of enigmatic musculoskeletal pain and dysfunction," Journal of Electromyography and Kinesiology, vol. 14, no. 1, pp. 95–107, 2004.

56. D. G. Simons, C. Z. Hong, and L. S. Simons, "Endplate potentials are common to midfiber myofacial trigger points," American Journal of Physical Medicine and Rehabilitation, vol. 81, no. 3, pp. 212–222, 2002.

57. D. G. Simons, C. Z. Hong, and L. S. Simons, "Prevalence of spontaneous electrical activity at trigger spots and at control sites in rabbit skeletal muscle," Journal of Musculoskeletal Pain, vol. 3, no. 1, pp. 35–48, 1995.

58. D. G. Simons, J. G. Travell, and L. S. Simons, Travell and Simons' Myofascial Pain and Dysfunction: The Trigger Point Manual, Lippincott Williams & Wilkins, Baltimore, Pa, USA, 2nd edition, 1999.

59. D. Gerwin, "Myofascial aspects of low back pain," Neurosurgery clinics of North America, vol. 2, no. 4, pp. 761–784, 1991.

60. D. Gerwin, "The taut band and other mysteries of the trigger point: an examination of the mechanisms relevant to the development and maintenance of the trigger point," Journal of Musculoskeletal Pain, vol. 16, no. 1-2, pp. 115–121, 2008.

61. D. Gerwin, J. Dommerholt, and J. P. Shah, "An expansion of Simons' integrated hypothesis of trigger point formation," Current Pain and Headache Reports, vol. 8, no. 6, pp. 468–475, 2004.

62. D. J. Webb, K. Donais, L. A. Whitmore et al., "FAK-Src signalling through paxillin, ERK and MLCK regulates adhesion disassembly," Nature Cell Biology, vol. 6, no. 2,pp. 154–161, 2004.

63. D. V. Nelson and D. M. Novy, "Psychological characteristics of reflex sympathetic dystrophy versus myofascial pain syndromes," Regional Anesthesia, vol. 21, no. 3, pp. 202–208, 1996.

64. D.G.Simons, C. Z.Hong, andL. S. Simons, "Endplatepotentials are common to midfiber myofacial trigger points," American Journal of Physical Medicine & Rehabilitation, vol. 81, no. 3, pp. 212–222, 2002.

65. Davies and Davies The Trigger Point Therapy Workbook second addition New Harbinger Publications CA, 2005

66. Dilorenzo L, Traballesi M, Morelli D, et al. Hemiparetic shoulder pain syndrome treated with deep dry needling during early rehabilitation: a prospective, open-label, randomized investigation. J Musculoskeletal Pain. 2004;12(2):25-34.

67. Doggweiler-Wiygul R. Urologic myofascial pain syndromes. Curr Pain Headache Rep. Dec 2004;8(6):445-451.

68. Dommerholt J, Moral O, Gröbli C. Trigger point dry needling. J Man Manip Ther. 2006;14(4):E70–87.

69. Dommerholt J, Stanborough RW. Muscle pain syndromes. In: Cantu RI, Grodin AJ, Stanborough RW, eds. Myofascial Manipulation. Austin: Pro-Ed; 2012:125-180.15 | Page

70. Dommerholt J. Complex regional pain syndrome; part 1: history, diagnostic criteria and etiology. J Bodywork Movement Ther. 2004;8(3):167-177.

71. Dommerholt J. Dry needling — peripheral and central considerations. J Manual Manipul Ther. 2011;19(4):223-237.

72. Dommerholt J. Persistent myalgia following whiplash. Curr Pain Headache Rep. Oct 2005;9(5):326-330.

73. Dommerholt, C. Bron, and J. Franssen, "Myofascial trigger points: an evidence-informed review," The Journal of Manual and ManipulativeTherapy, vol. 14, no. 4, pp. 203–221, 2006.

74. E. A. Tough, A. R. White, T. M. Cummings, S. H. Richards, and J. L. Campbell, "Acupuncture and dry needling in the management of myofascial trigger point pain: a systematic review and meta-analysis of randomised controlled trials," European Journal of Pain, vol. 13, no. 1, pp. 3–10, 2009.

75. E. Rios and G. Brum, "Involvement of dihydropyridine receptors in excitation-contraction coupling in skeletal muscle," Nature, vol. 325, no. 6106, pp. 717–720, 1987.

76. E. S. Pronker, T. C. Weenen, H. Commandeur, E. H. Claassen, andA.D.Osterhaus, "Risk in vaccine research and development quantified," PLoS ONE, vol. 8, no. 3, Article ID e57755, 2013.

77. E. S. Yang, P. W. Li, B. Nilius, and G. Li, "Ancient Chinese medicine and mechanistic evidence of acupuncture physiology," Pflügers Archiv, vol. 462, no. 5, pp. 645–653, 2011.

78. Edwards J, Knowles N. Superficial dry needling and active stretching in the treatment of myofascial pain--a randomised controlled trial. Acupunct Med. 2003/9 2003;21(3 SU):80-86.

79. Elorriaga A. The 2-Needle Technique. Med Acupunct. 2000;12(1):17-19.

80. Eto H, Suga H, Aci N, et al. Therapeutic potential of fibroblast growth factor-2 for hypertrophic scars: upregulation of MMP-1 and HGF expression. Lab Invest. Feb 2012;92(2):214-223.

81. Ettlin T, Schuster C, Stoffel R, Bruderlin A, Kischka U. A distinct pattern of myofascial findings in patients after whiplash injury. Arch Phys Med Rehabil. Jul 2008;89(7):1290-1293.

82. F. A. Araújo, M. A. Rocha, J. B. Mendes, and S. P. Andrade, "Atorvastatin inhibits inflammatory angiogenesis in mice through down regulation of VEGF, TNF-α and TGF-β1," Biomedicine and Pharmacotherapy, vol. 64, no. 1, pp. 29–34, 2010.

83. F. Kadi, K. Waling, C. Ahlgren et al., "Pathological mechanisms implicated in localized female trapezius myalgia," Pain, vol. 78, no. 3, pp. 191–196, 1998.

84. F. Lembeck and J. Donnerer, "Opioid control of the function of primary afferent substance P fibres,"European Journal of Pharmacology, vol. 114, no. 3, pp. 241–246, 1985.

85. Fernández de las Peñas C, Alonso Blanco C, Cuadrado ML, Pareja JA. Myofascial trigger points in the suboccipital muscles in episodic tension-type headache. Man Ther. 2006;11:225-230.14 | Page

86. Fernández de las Peñas C, Cuadrado M, Arendt-Nielsen L, Simons D, Pareja J. Myofascial trigger points and sensitization: an updated pain model for tension-type headache. Cephalalgia. 2007;27(5):383-393.11 | Page

87. Fernández de las Peñas C, Ge HY, Arendt-Nielsen L, Cuadrado ML, Pareja JA. The local and referred pain from myofascial trigger points in the temporalis muscle contributes to pain profile in chronic tension-type headache. Clin J Pain. Nov-Dec 2007;23(9):786-792.

88. Fernández de las Peñas CF, Cuadrado ML, Gerwin RD, Pareja JA. Referred pain from the trochlear region in tension-type headache: a myofascial trigger point from the superior oblique muscle. Headache. Jun 2005;45(6):731-737.

89. Fernández-Carnero J, Fernández de las Peñas CF, de la Llave-Rincón AI, Ge HY, Arendt-Nielsen L. Prevalence of and referred pain from myofascial trigger points in the forearm muscles in patients with lateral epicondylalgia. Clin J Pain. May 2007;23(4):353-360.

90. Fernández-de-las-Peñas C, Ge HY, Alonso-Blanco C, González-Iglesias J, Arendt-Nielsen L. Referred pain areas of active myofascial trigger points in head, neck, and shoulder muscles, in chronic tension type headache. J Bodyw Mov Ther. Oct 2010;14(4):391-396.

91. Findley TW. Fascia Research from a Clinician/Scientist's Perspective. Int JTher Massage Bodywork. 2011;4(4):1-6.

92. Freeman MD, Nystrom A, Centeno C. Chronic whiplash and central sensitization; an evaluation of the role of a myofascial trigger points in pain modulation. J Brachial Plex Peripher Nerve Inj. 2009;4:2.

93. Fricton JR. Etiology and management of masticatory myofascial pain. J Musculoskeletal Pain. 1999;7(1/2):143-160.

94. Fruth SJ. Differential diagnosis and treatment in a patient with posterior upper thoracic pain. Phys Ther Feb 2006;86(2):254-268.

95. Fu ZH, Chen XY, Lu LJ, Lin J, Xu JG. Immediate effect of Fu's subcutaneous needling for low back pain. Chin Med J. (Engl). Jun 5 2006;119(11):953-956.

96. Fu ZH, Wang JH, Sun JH, Chen XY, Xu JG. Fu's subcutaneous needling: possible clinical evidence of the subcutaneous connective tissue in acupuncture. J Altern Complement Med. Jan-Feb 2007;13(1):47-51.

97. G. Loor and P. T. Schumacker, "Role of hypoxia-inducible factor in cell survival during myocardial ischemia-reperfusion," Cell Death and Differentiation, vol. 15, no. 4, pp. 686–690, 2008.

98. G. S. Supinski and L. A. Callahan, "Free radical-mediated skeletal muscle dysfunction in inflammatory conditions," Journal of Applied Physiology, vol. 102, no. 5, pp. 2056–2063, 2007.

99. G. S. Supinski, H. Bark, A. Guanciale, and S. G. Kelsen, "Effect of alterations in muscle fiber length on diaphragmblood flow," Journal of Applied Physiology, vol. 60, no. 5, pp. 1789–1796, 1986.

100. Ga H, Choi JH, Park CH, Yoon HJ. Dry needling of trigger points with and without paraspinal needling in myofascial pain syndromes in elderly patients. J Altern Complement Med. 2007;13 (6):617–24.

101. Ge HY, Fernandez-de-Las-Penas C, Yue SW. Myofascial trigger points: spontaneous electrical activity and its consequences for pain induction and propagation. Chinese Medicine. 2011;6:13.

102. Gerwin RD, Dommerholt J, Shah JP. An expansion of Simons' integrated hypothesis of trigger point formation. Curr Pain Headache Rep. Dec 2004;8(6):468-475.

103. Gerwin RD, Dommerholt J. Treatment of myofascial pain syndromes. In: Boswell MV, Cole BE, eds. Weiner's pain management; a practical guide for clinicians. Vol 7. Boca Raton: CRC Press; 2006:477-492.

104. Giamberardino MA, Tafuri E, Savini A, et al. Contribution of myofascial trigger points to migraine symptoms. J Pain. Nov 2007;8(11):869-878.

105. Gissel, "The role of Ca2+ in muscle cell damage," Annals of the New York Academy of Sciences, vol. 1066, pp. 166–180, 2005.

106. Graven-Nielsen T, Babenko V, Svensson P, Arendt-Nielsen L. Experimentally induced muscle pain induces hypoalgesia in heterotopic deep tissues, but not in homotopic deep tissues. Brain Res. 1998;787(2):203–10.

107. Grinnell F. Fibroblast biology in three-dimensional collagen matrices. Trends Cell Biol. May 2003;13(5):264-269.

108. Guerreiro da Silva AV, Uchiyama Nakamura M, Guerreiro da Silva JB. 'Forbidden points' in pregnancy: do they exist? Acupunct Med. 2011;29:135–136.

109. H. Gerber, S. Sikdar, K. Armstrong et al., "A systematic comparison between subjects with no pain and pain associated with active myofascial trigger points," PM & R: The Journal of 12 International Scholarly Research Notices Injury, Function, and Rehabilitation, vol. 5, no. 11, pp. 931–938, 2013.

110. H. Hoppeler, O. Mathieu, R. Krauer, H. Claassen, R. B. Armstrong, and E. R.Weibel, "Design of themammalian respiratory system. VI. Distribution of mitochondria and capillaries in various muscles," Respiration Physiology vol. 44, no. 1, pp. 87–111, 1981.

111. H. J. Lee, J. H. Lee, E. O. Lee et al., "Substance P and beta endorphin mediate electroacupuncture induced analgesic activity in mouse cancer pain model," Acupuncture & Electro-Therapeutics Research, vol. 34, no. 1-2, pp. 27–40, 2009.

112. H. Tsutsui, S. Kinugawa, and S. Matsushima, "Oxidative stress and heart failure," American Journal of Physiology: Heart and Circulatory Physiology, vol. 301, no. 6, pp. H2181–H2190, 2011.

113. H. Y. Ge, "Prevalence of myofascial trigger points in fibromyalgia:the overlap of two common problems," Current Pain and Headache Reports, vol. 14, no. 5, pp. 339–345, 2010.

114. H. Y. Ge, L. Arendt-Nielsen, and P. Madeleine, "Accelerated muscle fatigability of latent myofascial trigger points in humans," Pain Medicine, vol. 13, no. 7, pp. 957–964, 2012.

115. H.Ga, H. J. Koh, J. H. Choi, andC. H. Kim, "Intramuscular and nerve root stimulation vs lidocaine: injection to trigger points in myofascial pain syndrome," Journal of Rehabilitation Medicine, vol. 39, no. 5, pp. 374–378, 2007.

116. H.-Y. Ge, C. Fern'andez-de-las-Pe~nas, and S.-W. Yue, "Myofascial trigger points: spontaneous electrical activity and its consequences for pain induction and propagation," ChineseMedicine, vol. 6, article 13, 2011.

117. Hicks MR, Cao TV, Campbell DH, Standley PR. Mechanical strain applied to human fibroblasts differentially regulates skeletal myoblast differentiation. J Appl Physiol. Aug 2012;113(3):465-472.

118. Hidalgo-Lozano, C. Fern'andez-de-las-Pe~nas, C. Calder'on- Soto, A. Domingo-Camara, P. Madeleine, and M. Arroyo- Morales, "Elite swimmers with and without unilateral shoulder pain: mechanical hyperalgesia and active/latent muscle trigger points in neck-shoulder muscles," Scandinavian Journal of Medicine and Science in Sports, vol. 23, no. 1, pp. 66–73, 2013.

119. Hinz B, Phan SH, Thannickal VJ, et al. Recent developments in myofibroblast biology: paradigms for connective tissue remodeling. Am J Pathol. Apr 2012;180(4):1340-1355.

120. Hinz B. The myofibroblast: paradigm for a mechanically active cell. J Biomech. Jan 5 2010;43(1):146-155.

121. Hong C-Z, Chen Y-N, Twehous D, Hong D H Pressure threshold for referred pain by compression on the trigger point and adjacent areas. Journal of Musculoskeletal Pain 4(3): 61–79 1996

122. Hong CZ, Kuan TS, Chen JT, Chen SM. Referred pain elicited by palpation and by needling of myofascial trigger points: a comparison. Arch Phys Med Rehabil. 1997;78(9):957-960.

123. Hong CZ, Simons DG. Pathophysiologic and electrophysiologic mechanisms of myofascial trigger points. Arch Phys Med Rehabil. 1998;79(7):863-872.

124. Hong CZ, Torigoe Y, Yu J. The localized twitch responses in responsive bands of rabbit skeletal muscle are related to the reflexes at spinal cord level. J Muscoskel Pain. 1995;3:15-33.

125. Hong C-Z, Yu J. Spontaneous electrical activity of rabbit trigger spot after transection of spinal cord and peripheral nerve. J Musculoskelet Pain. 1998;6(4):45-58.

126. Hong CZ. Lidocaine injection versus dry needling to myofascial trigger point. The importance of the local twitch response. Am J Phys Med Rehabil. 1994;73(4):256-263.

127. Hong CZ. Lidocaine injection versus dry needling to myofascial trigger point. The importance of the local twitch response. Am J Phys Med Rehabil. 1994;73(4):256–63.

128. Hong CZ. Persistence of local twitch response with loss of conduction to and from the spinal cord. Arch Phys Med Rehabil. Jan 1994;75(1):12-16.

129. Hong, C.Z.. Lidocaine injection versus Dry Needling to myofascial trigger point. The importance of the local twitch response. American Journal of Physical Medicine and Rehabilitation 73:256-263,1994b

130. Hoyle JA, Marras WS, Sheedy JE, Hart DE. Effects of postural and visual stressors on myofascialtrigger point development and motor unit rotation during computer work. J Electromyogr Kinesiol. Feb 2011;21(1):41-48.

131. Hsieh YL, Chou LW, Joe YS, Hong CZ. Spinal cord mechanism involving the remote effects of dry needling on the irritability of myofascial trigger spots in rabbit skeletal muscle. Arch Phys Med Rehabil. Jul 2011;92(7):1098-1105.

132. Hsieh YL, Chou LW, Joe YS, Hong CZ. Spinal cord mechanism involving the remote effects of dry needling on the irritability of myofascial trigger spots in rabbit skeletal muscle. Arch Phys Med Rehabil. 2011;92(7):1098–105.

133. Hsueh TC, Yu S, Kuan TS, Hong CZ. Association of active myofascial trigger points and cervical disc lesions. J Formos Med Assoc. 1998;97(3):174-180.

134. http://neuroscience.uth.tmc.edu/s3/chapter01.html accessed 12/14/12; Figure 1: http://basic-clinical-pharmacology.net (accessed 12/15/12)

135. http://www.maherpt.com/IMT.aspx (accessed 12/14/12) Figure 6: Reflex arc: Howard Fields' Pain, McGraw Hill 1987. Figure 7: spray and stretch www.bodyreliefdepot.com (accessed 12/15/12)

136. Huang YT, Lin SY, Neoh CA, Wang KY, Jean YH, Shi HY. Dry needling for myofascial pain: prognostic factors. J Altern Complement Med. 2011;17(8):755–62.

137. Huguenin L, Brukner PD, McCrory P, Smith P, Wajswelner H, Bennell K. Effect of dry needling of gluteal muscles on straight leg raise: a randomised, placebo controlled, double blind trial. Br J Sports Med. 2005;39(2):84–90.

138. I. Flinder, O. A. Timofeeva, C. M. Rosseland, L. Wierød, H. S. Huitfeldt, and E. Skarpen, "EGF-induced ERK-activation downstream of FAK requires rac1-NADPH oxidase," Journal of Cellular Physiology, vol. 226, no. 9, pp. 2267–2278, 2011.

139. In this study, the effects of remote dry needling appear to be associated with the activation of the diffuse noxious inhibitory control system. This has importance for treating those patients who are too sensitive for direct needling of involved muscles.

140. Iqbal SA, Sidgwick GP, Bayat A. Identification of fibrocytes from mesenchymal stem cells in keloid tissue: a potential source of abnormal fibroblasts in keloid scarring. Arch. Dermatol Res. Oct 2012;304(8):665-671.

141. Itoh K, Minakawa Y, Kitakoji H. Effect of acupuncture depth on muscle pain. Chin Med. 2011;6(1):24.

142. J. Chiang, Y. C. Shen, Y. H. Wang et al., "Honokiol protects rats against eccentric exercise-induced skeletal muscle damage by inhibiting NF-κB induced oxidative stress and inflammation," European Journal of Pharmacology, vol. 610, no. 1–3, pp. 119–127, 2009.

143. J. Fleckenstein, D. Zaps, L. J. R¨uger et al., "Discrepancy between prevalence and perceived effectiveness of treatment methods in myofascial pain syndrome: results of a cross-sectional, nationwide survey," BMC Musculoskeletal Disorders, vol. 11, article 32, 2010.

144. J. Jarrell, "Myofascial pain in the adolescent," Current Opinion in Obstetrics and Gynecology, vol. 22, no. 5, pp. 393–398, 2010.

145. J. P. Shah and E. A. Gilliams, "Uncovering the biochemical milieu of myofascial trigger points using in vivo microdialysis: an application of muscle pain concepts to myofascial pain syndrome," Journal of Bodywork and Movement Therapies, vol. 12, no. 4, pp. 371–384, 2008.

146. J. P. Shah and E. A. Gilliams, "Uncovering the biochemical milieu of myofascial trigger points using in vivo microdialysis: an application of muscle pain concepts to myofascial pain syndrome," Journal of Bodywork and Movement Therapies, vol. 12, no. 4, pp. 371–384, 2008.

147. J. P. Shah, J. V. Danoff, M. J. Desai et al., "Biochemicals associated with pain and inflammation are elevated in sites near to and remote from active myofascial trigger points," Archives of Physical Medicine and Rehabilitation, vol. 89, no. 1, pp. 16–23, 2008.

148. J. R. Fricton, M. D. Auvinen, D. Dykstra, and E. Schiffman, "Myofascial pain syndrome. Electromyographic changes associated with local twitch response," Archives of Physical Medicine and Rehabilitation, vol. 66, no. 5, pp. 314–317, 1985.

149. J. Rein¨ohl, U. Hoheisel, T. Unger, and S. Mense, "Adenosine triphosphate as a stimulant for nociceptive and non-nociceptive muscle group IV receptors in the rat," Neuroscience Letters, vol. 338, no. 1, pp. 25–28, 2003.

150. J. T. Liou, F. C. Liu, C. C. Mao, Y. S. Lai, and Y. J. Day, "Inflammation confers dual effects on nociceptive processing in chronic neuropathic pain model," Anesthesiology, vol. 114, no. 3, pp. 660–672, 2011.

151. Jaeger, "Myofascial trigger point pain," The Alpha Omegan, vol. 106, no. 1-2, pp. 14–22, 2013.

152. Jarrell J. Myofascial dysfunction in the pelvis. Curr Pain Headache Rep. Dec 2004;8(6):452-456.

153. Jarrell JF, Vilos GA, Allaire C, et al. Consensus guidelines for the management of chronic pelvic pain. J Obstet Gynaecol Can. Sept 2005;27(9):869-887.

154. K. H. Chen, C. Z. Hong, F. C. Kuo, H. C. Hsu, and Y. L. Hsieh, "Electrophysiologic effects of a therapeutic laser on myofascial trigger spots of rabbit skeletal muscles," American Journal of Physical Medicine and Rehabilitation, vol. 87, no. 12, pp. 1006–1014, 2008.

155. K. H. Chen, C. Z. Hong, H. C. Hsu, S. K. Wu, F. C. Kuo, and Y. L. Hsieh, "Dose-dependent and ceiling effects of therapeutic laser on myofascial trigger spots in rabbit skeletal muscles," Journal of Musculoskeletal Pain, vol. 18, no. 3, pp. 235–245, 2010.

156. K. Powers and M. J. Jackson, "Exercise-induced oxidative stress: cellularmechanisms and impact onmuscle force production," Physiological Reviews, vol. 88, no. 4, pp. 1243–1276, 2008.

157. K. Powers, W. B. Nelson, and M. B. Hudson, "Exerciseinduced oxidative stress in humans: cause and consequences," Free Radical Biology and Medicine, vol. 51, no. 5, pp. 942–950, 2011.

158. K. Sakellariou, A. Vasilaki, J. Palomero et al., "Studies of mitochondrial and nonmitochondrial sources implicate nicotinamide adenine dinucleotide phosphate oxidase(s) in the increased skeletal muscle superoxide generation that occurs during contractile activity," Antioxidants and Redox Signaling, vol. 18, no. 6, pp. 603–621, 2013.

159. K. Schwerzmann, H. Hoppeler, S. R. Kayar, and E. R. Weibel, "Oxidative capacity of muscle and mitochondria: correlation of physiological, biochemical, and morphometric characteristics," Proceedings of the National Academy of Sciences of the United States of America, vol. 86, no. 5, pp. 1583–1587, 1989.

160. K. Tang, E. C. Breen, H. Wagner, T. D. Brutsaert, M. Gassmann, and P. D. Wagner, "HIF and VEGF relationships in response to hypoxia and sciatic nerve stimulation in rat gastrocnemius," Respiratory Physiology and Neurobiology, vol. 144, no. 1, pp. 71–80, 2004.

161. Kalichman L, Vulfsons S. Dry needling in the management of musculoskeletal pain. J Am Board Fam Med. 2010;23(5):640-6.

162. Kamanli A, Kaya A, Ardicoglu O, Ozgocmen S, Zengin FO, Bayik Y. Comparison of lidocaine injection, botulinum toxin injection, and dry needling to trigger points in myofascial pain syndrome. Rheumatol Int. 2005;25(8):604–11.

163. Kennedy B, Beckert L. A case of acupuncture-induced pneumothorax. N Z Med J. 2010;123(1320):88–90.

164. Kern KU, Martin C, Scheicher S, Muller H. Auslosung von Phantomschmerzen und –sensationen durch muskulare Stumpftriggerpunkte nach Beinamputationen [Referred pain from amputation stump trigger points into the phantom limb]. Schmerz. Aug 2006;20(4):300-306.

165. Kern U, Martin C, Scheicher S, Müller H. Does botulinum toxin A make prosthesis use easier for amputees? J Rehabil Med. Sep 2004;36(5):238-239.

166. Khan KM, Scott A. Mechanotherapy: how physical therapists' prescription of exercise promotes tissue repair. Br J Sports Med. Apr 2009;43(4):247-252.

167. Knierim J. Pain modulation and mechanisms. [Online]. The University of Texas Health Science Center at Houston. http://neuroscience.uth.tmc.edu/s2/chapter08.html [12/19/12].

168. Kraft G H, Johnson E W, La Ban M M The fibrositis syndrome. Archives of Physical Medicine and Rehabilitation 49: 155–1621963

169. Kuan TS, Hsieh YL, Chen SM, Chen JT, Yen WC, Hong CZ. The myofascial trigger point region: correlation between the degree of irritability and the prevalence of endplate noise. Am J Phys Med Rehabil. 2007;86(3):183-189.

170. L. Hordijk, "Regulation of NADPH oxidases: the role of Rac proteins," Circulation Research, vol. 98, no. 4, pp. 453–462, 2006.

171. L. I. Filippin, A. J. Moreira, N. P. Marroni, and R. M. Xavier, "Nitric oxide and repair of skeletal muscle injury," Nitric Oxide, vol. 21, no. 3-4, pp. 157–163, 2009.

172. L. Kalichman and S. Vulfsons, "Dry needling in the management of musculoskeletal pain," Journal of the American Board of Family Medicine, vol. 23, no. 5, pp. 640–646, 2010.

173. L. P. Michaelson, G. Shi, C. W. Ward, and G. G. Rodney, "Mitochondrial redox potential during contraction in single intact muscle fibers," Muscle & Nerve, vol. 42, no. 4, pp. 522–529, 2010.

174. L. Post, S. M. Sarracino, S. D. Gergis, and M. D. Sokoll, "Comparative effects of etidocaine and lidocaine on nerve and neuromuscular conduction in the frog," Acta Anaesthesiologica Scandinavica, vol. 26, no. 5, pp. 463–467, 1982.

175. L. Rosendal, B. Larsson, J. Kristiansen et al., "Increase in muscle nociceptive substances and anaerobic metabolism in patients with trapezius myalgia: microdialysis in rest and during exercise," Pain, vol. 112, no. 3, pp. 324–334, 2004.

176. L. Tekin, S. Akarsu, O. Durmuş, E. Cakar, U. Dinçer, and M. Z. Kıralp, "The effect of dry needling in the treatment of myofascial pain syndrome: a randomized double-blinded placebo-controlled trial," Clinical Rheumatology. In press.

177. L. W. Chou, Y. L. Hsieh, M. J. Kao, and C. Z. Hong, "Remote influences of acupuncture on the pain intensity and the amplitude changes of endplate noise in the myofascial trigger point of the upper trapezius muscle," Archives of Physical Medicine and Rehabilitation, vol. 90, no. 6, pp. 905–912, 2009.

178. Langevin HM, Bouffard NA, Badger GJ, Churchill DL, Howe AK. Subcutaneous tissue fibroblast cytoskeletal remodeling induced by acupuncture: Evidence for a mechanotransduction-based mechanism. J Cell Physiol. May 2006;207(3):767-774.

179. Langevin HM, Bouffard NA, Badger GJ, Iatridis JC, Howe AK. Dynamic fibroblast cytoskeletal response to subcutaneous tissue stretch ex vivo and in vivo. Am J Physiol Cell Physiol. Mar 2005;288(3):C747-756.

180. Langevin HM, Bouffard NA, Fox JR, et al. Fibroblast cytoskeletal remodeling contributes to connective tissue tension. J Cell Physiol. May 2011;226(5):1166-1175.

181. Langevin HM, Churchill DL, Cipolla MJ. Mechanical signaling through connective tissue: a mechanism for the therapeutic effect of acupuncture. FASEB J. Oct 2001;15(12):2275-2282.

182. Langevin HM, Storch KN, Snapp RR, et al. Tissue stretch induces nuclear remodeling in connective tissue fibroblasts. Histochem Cell Biol. Apr 2010;133(4):405-415.

183. Lee JH, Lee H, Jo DJ. An acute cervical epidural hematoma as a complication of dry needling. Spine (Phila Pa 1976). 2011;36(13): E891–3.

184. Lee WM, Leung HB, Wong WC. Iatrogenic bilateral pneumothorax arising from acupuncture: a case report. J Orthop Surg (Hong Kong). 2005;13(3):300–2.

185. Legrain V, Iannetti GD, Plaghki L, Mouraux A. The pain matrix reloaded: a salience detection system for the body. Prog Neurobiol. Jan 2011;93(1):111-124.

186. Lewit K, Olsanska S. Clinical importance of active scars: abnormal scars as a cause of myofascial pain. J Manipulative Physiol Ther. 2004;27(6):399-402.

187. Longbottom J. A case report of postulated 'Barré Liéou syndrome'. Acupunct Med. Mar 2005;23(1):34-38.

188. Lucas KR, Polus BI, Rich PS. Latent myofascial trigger points: their effects on muscle activation and movement efficiency. J Bodyw Mov Ther. 2004;8:160-166.

189. Lucas KR, Rich PA, Polus BI. Muscle activation patterns in the scapular positioning muscles during loaded scapular plane elevation: the effects of latent myofascial trigger points. Clin Biomechanics. 2010;25(8):765-770.

190. Lundeberg T, Lund I. Is there a role for acupuncture in endometriosis pain, or 'endometrialgia'? Acupunct Med. Jun 2008;26(2):94-110.

191. M. Bergeron, A. Y. Yu, K. E. Solway, G. L. Semenza, and F. R. Sharp, "Induction of hypoxia-inducible factor-1 (HIF-1) and its target genes following focal ischaemia in rat brain," European Journal of Neuroscience, vol. 11, no. 12, pp. 4159–4170, 1999.

192. M. C. Gong, S. Arbogast, Z. Guo, J. Mathenia, W. Su, and M. B. Reid, "Calcium-independent phospholipase A2 modulates cytosolic oxidant activity and contractile function in murine skeletalmuscle cells," Journal of Applied Physiology, vol. 100, no. 2, pp. 399–405, 2006.

193. M. Capes, R. Loaiza, and H. H. Valdivia, "Ryanodine receptors," Skeletal Muscle, vol. 1, no. 1, article 18, 2011.

194. M. Gomez-Cabrera, C. Borr'as, F. V. Pallardo, J. Sastre, L. L. Ji, and J. Vi~na, "Decreasing xanthine oxidase-mediated oxidative stress prevents useful cellular adaptations to exercise in rats," The Journal of Physiology, vol. 567, no. 1, pp. 113–120, 2005.

195. M. Hopkins, "Skeletalmuscle physiology," Continuing Education in Anaesthesia, Critical Care and Pain, vol. 6, no. 1, pp. 1–6, 2006.

196. M. J. Jackson, "Control of reactive oxygen species production in contracting skeletal muscle," Antioxidants and Redox Signaling, vol. 15, no. 9, pp. 2477–2486, 2011.

197. M. Milkiewicz and T. L. Haas, "Effect of mechanical stretch on HIF-1α and MMP-2 expression in capillaries isolated from overloaded skeletal muscles: laser capture microdissection study," American Journal of Physiology, vol. 289, no. 3, pp. H1315–H1320, 2005.

198. M. S. Jafri, S. J. Dudycha, and B. O'Rourke, "Cardiac energy metabolism: models of cellular respiration," Annual Review of Biomedical Engineering, vol. 3, pp. 57–81, 2001.

199. M. Schrier, D. Amital, Y. Arnson et al., "Association of fibromyalgia characteristics in patients with non-metastatic breast cancer and the protective role of resilience," Rheumatology International, vol. 32, no. 10, pp. 3017–3023, 2012.

200. M. Zimmermann, "Ethical considerations in relation to pain in animal experimentation," Acta Physiologica Scandinavica, vol. 128, no. 554, pp. 221–233, 1986.

201. M. Zimmermann, "Ethical guidelines for investigations of experimental pain in conscious animals,"Pain, vol. 16, no. 2, pp 109–110, 1983.

202. Majlesi J, Unalan H. Effect of treatment on trigger points. Curr Pain Headache Rep. Oct 2010;14(5):353-360.

203. Mayoral O, De Felipe JA, Martínez JM. Changes in tenderness and tissue compliance in myofascial trigger points with a new technique of electroacupuncture. Three preliminary cases report. J Muscoskel Pain. 2004;12(suppl):33.

204. McCutcheon LJ, Yelland M. Iatrogenic pneumothorax: safety concerns when using acupuncture or dry needling in the thoracic region. Phys Ther Rev. 2011;16(2):126–32.

205. McPartland JM, Simons DG. Myofascial trigger points: translating molecular theory into manual therapy. J Man Manipulative Ther. 2006;14(4):232-239.

206. McPartland JM. Expression of the endocannabinoid system in fibroblasts and myofascial tissues. J Bodyw Mov Ther. Apr 2008;12(2):169-182.

207. Mense S. How do muscle lesions such as latent and active trigger points influence central nociceptive neurons? J Muscu okelet Pain. 2010;18(4):348-353.

208. Mense S. Morphology of myofascial trigger points: what does a trigger point look like? In: Mense S, Gerwin R, D., eds. Muscle pain; diagnosis and treatment. Heidelberg: Springer; 2010:85-102.

209. Mitchell, "Coupling of phosphorylation to electron and hydrogen transfer by a chemi-osmotic type of mechanism," Nature, vol. 191, no. 4784, pp. 144–148, 1961.

210. Moseley GL. A pain neuromatrix approach to patients with chronic pain. Man Ther. Sep 2003;8(3):130-140.

211. N.Akkaya, N. S. Atalay, S.T. Selcuk, H. Alkan, N. Catalbas, and F. Sahin, "Frequency of fibromyalgia syndrome in breast cancer patients," International Journal of Clinical Oncology vol. 18, no. 2, pp. 285–292, 2013.

212. National Centers for Health Statistics, Chartbook on Trends in the Health of Americans 2006. Special Feature: Pain. http://www.cdc.gov/nchs/data/hus/hus06.pdf. (accessed 12/17/12)

213. Nicholls JG, Martin AR, Wallace BG, Fuchs PA. From Neuron to Brain. 4th ed. Massachusetts: Sinauer Associates, Inc., 2001.

214. Niddam DM, Chan RC, Lee SH, Yeh TC, Hsieh JC. Central modulation of pain evoked from myofascial trigger point. Clin J Pain. Jun 2007;23(5):440-448.

215. Niddam DM, Chan RC, Lee SH, Yeh TC, Hsieh JC. Central modulation of pain evoked from myofascial trigger point. Clin J Pain. 2007;23(5):440–8.

216. Niddam DM, Chan RC, Lee SH, Yeh TC, Hsieh JC. Central representation of hyperalgesia from myofascial trigger point. Neuroimage. Feb 1 2008;39(3):1299-1306.

217. Olausson H, Lamarre Y, Backlund H, et al. Unmyelinated tactile afferents signal touch and project to insular cortex. Nat Neurosci Sep 2002;5(9):900-904.

218. P. L. Wood, "Animal models in analgesic testing," in Central Nervous System Pharmacology. Analgesics: Neurochemical, Behavioral and Clinical Perspective, M. J. Kuhar and G. W. Pasternak, Eds., pp. 175–194. Raven Press, New York, NY, USA, 1984.

219. P.E. Baldry, John W. ThompsonAcupuncture, Trigger Points and Musculoskeletal Pain (Third Edition), 2005, Pages 73-100; Figure 2: Baldry, John W. ThompsonAcupuncture, Trigger Points and Musculoskeletal Pain (Third Edition), 2005, Pages 74, figure 7.1 P.E.

220. Pérez-Palomares S, Oliván-Blázquez B, Magallón-Botaya R, et al. Percutaneous electrical nerve stimulation versus dry needling: effectiveness in the treatment of chronic low back pain. J Musculoskelet Pain. 2010;18(1):23–30.

221. Peuker ET, White A, Ernst E, Pera F, Filler TJ. Traumatic complications of acupuncture. Therapists need to know human anatomy. Arch Fam Med. 1999;8(6):553–8.

222. Prateepavanich P, Kupniratsaikul V, Charoensak T. The relationship between myofascial trigger points of gastrocnemius muscle and nocturnal calf cramps. J Med Assoc Thailand. 1999;82:451- 459.

223. Q. Fang Li, H. Xu, Y. Sun, R. Hu, and H. Jiang, "Induction of inducible nitric oxide synthase by isoflurane post-conditioning via hypoxia inducible factor-1α during tolerance against ischemic neuronal injury," Brain Research, vol. 1451, pp. 1–9, 2012.

224. Qerama E, Kasch H, Fuglsang-Frederiksen A. Occurrence of myofascial pain in patients with possible carpal tunnel syndrome - a single-blinded study. Eur J Pain. Jul 2009;13(6):588-591.

225. R. A. Mesquita-Ferrari, M. D. Martins, J. A. Silva Jr. et al., "Effects of low-level laser therapy on expression of TNF-α and TGF-β in skeletal muscle during the repair process," Lasers in Medical Science, vol. 26, no. 3, pp. 335–340, 2011.

226. R. S. Fitzgerald, M. Shirahata, and I. Chang, "The impact of PCO2 and H+ on the release of acetylcholine from the cat carotid body," Neuroscience Letters, vol. 397, no. 3, pp. 205–209, 2006.

227. R. Sekido, K. Ishimaru, and M. Sakita, "Differences of electroacupuncture-induced analgesic effect in normal and inflammatory conditions in rats," American Journal of Chinese Medicine, vol. 31, no. 6, pp. 955–965, 2003.

228. R. Taguchi, T. Taguchi, and H. Kitakoji, "Involvement of peripheral opioid receptors in electroacupuncture analgesia for carrageenan-induced hyperalgesia," Brain Research, vol. 1355, pp. 97–103, 2010.

229. Rashiq S, Galer BS. Proximal myofascial dysfunction in complex regional pain syndrome: a retrospective prevalence study. Clin J Pain. Jun 1999;15(2):151-153.

230. Reinert A, Treede R, Bromm B. The pain inhibiting pain effect: an electrophysiological study in humans. Brain Res. 2000;862(1–2):103–10.

231. Rha DW, Shin JC, Kim YK, Jung JH, Kim YU, Lee SC. Detecting local twitch responses of myofascial trigger points in the lower-back muscles using ultrasonography. Arch Phys Med Rehabil. Oct 2011;92(10):1576-1580 e1571.

232. Rosomoff HL, Fishbain DA, Goldberg N, Rosomoff RS. Myofascial findings with patients with "chronic intractable benign pain: of the back and neck. Pain Management. 1989;3:114-118.

233. S. E. Larsson, L. Bodegard, K. G. Henriksson, and P. A. Oberg, "Chronic trapezius myalgia: morphology and blood flow studied in 17 patients," Acta Orthopaedica Scandinavica, vol. 61, no. 5, pp. 394–398, 1990.

234. S. Mense and D. G. Simons, Muscle Pain: Understanding Its Nature, Diagnosis, and Treatment, Philadelphia, Pa, USA, Lippincott Williams & Wilkins edition, 2001.

235. S. T. Russell, H. Eley, and M. J. Tisdale, "Role of reactive oxygen species in protein degradation in murine myotubes induced by proteolysis-inducing factor and angiotensin II," Cellular Signalling, vol. 19, no. 8, pp. 1797–1806, 2007.

236. Saladin KS. Anatomy & Physiology: The Unity of Form and Function. 5th ed. New York: McGraw-Hill, 2010.

237. Samuels ER, Szabadi E. Functional Neuroanatomy of the Noradrenergic Locus Coeruleus: Its Roles in the Regulation of Arousal and Autonomic Function Part I: Principles of Functional Organization. [Online] PubMed Central. http://www.ncbi.nlm.nih.gov/pmc/articles/PMC2687936/. [12/16/12].

238. Shah J, Phillips T, Danoff JV, Gerber LH. A novel microanalytical technique for assaying soft tissue demonstrates significant quantitative biomechanical differences in 3 clinically distinct groups: normal, latent and active. Arch Phys Med Rehabil. 2003;84:A4.

239. Shah JP, Danoff JV, Desai MJ, et al. Biochemicals associated with pain and inflammation are elevated in sites near to and remote from active myofascial trigger points. Arch Phys Med Rehabil. Jan 2008;89(1):16-23.

240. Shah JP, Gilliams EA. Uncovering the biochemical milieu of myofascial trigger points using in vivo microdialysis: an application of muscle pain concepts to myofascial pain syndrome. J Bodyw Mov Ther. Oct 2008;12(4):371-384.

241. Shah JP, Phillips TM, Danoff JV, Gerber LH. An in vivo microanalytical technique for measuring the local biochemical milieu of human skeletal muscle. J Appl Physiol. 2005;99(5):1977–84.

242. Shah JP, Phillips TM, Danoff JV, Gerber LH. An in-vivo microanalytical technique for measuring the local biochemical milieu of human skeletal muscle. J Appl Physiol. 2005;99:1977-1984.

243. Sikdar S, Shah JP, Gebreab T, et al. Novel applications of ultrasound technology to visualize and characterize myofascial trigger points and surrounding soft tissue. Arch Phys Med Rehabil. Nov 2009;90(11):1829-1838.

244. Sikdar S, Shah JP, Gebreab T, et al. Novel applications of ultrasound technology to visualize and characterize myofascial trigger points and surrounding soft tissue. Arch Phys Med Rehabil 2009;90(11):1829–38.

245. Simons D G Clinical and etiological update of myofascial pain from trigger points. Journal of Musculoskeletal pain 4(1/2): 93–121 1996

246. Simons D. Muscular pain syndrome. In: Friction J, Awad EA, editors. Advances in pain research and therapy. New York: Raven; 1990. p. 1–41.

247. Simons DG, Dexter JR. Comparison of local twitch responses elicited by palpation and needling of myofascial trigger points. J Musculoskeletal Pain. 1995;3:49-61.

248. Simons DG, Hong C-Z, Simons LS. Endplate potentials are common to midfiber myofascial trigger points. Am J Phys Med Rehabil. 2002;81(3):212-222.

249. Simons DG, Mense S. Understanding and measurement of muscle tone as related to clinical muscle pain. Pain. 1998;75(1):1-17.

250. Simons DG. New views of myofascial trigger points: etiology and diagnosis. Arch Phys Med Rehabil Jan 2008;89(1):157-159.

251. Simons DG. Review of enigmatic MTrPs as a common cause of enigmatic musculoskeletal pain and dysfunction. J Electromyogr Kinesiol. 2004;14:95-107.

252. Simons DG. Understanding effective treatments of myofascial trigger points. J Bodyw Mov Ther. 2002;6(2):81-88.

253. Sirker, M. Zhang, and A. M. Shah, "NADPH oxidases in cardiovascular disease: Insights from in vivo models and clinical studies," Basic Research in Cardiology, vol. 106, no. 5, pp. 735–747, 2011.

254. Skubick DL, Clasby R, Donaldson CC, Marshall WM. Carpal tunnel syndrome as an expression of muscular dysfunction in the neck. J Occupational Rehab. 1993;3(1):31-43.

255. Skutek M, van Griensven M. Zeichen J, Brauer N, Bosch U. Cyclic mechanical stretching enhances secretion of Interleukin 6 in human tendon fibroblasts. Knee Surg Sports Traumatol Arthrosc. Sep 2001;9(5):322-326.

256. Skutek M, van Griensven M. Zeichen J, Brauer N, Bosch U. Cyclic mechanical stretching modulates secretion pattern of growth factors in human tendon fibroblasts. Eur J Appl Physiol. Nov 2001;86(1):48-52

257. Squire LR, Bloom FE, McConnell SK, Roberts JL, Spitzer NC, Zigmond MJ. Fundamental Neuroscience. Florida: Elsevier Science, 2003.

258. Srbely JZ, Dickey JP, Lee D, Lowerison M. Dry needle stimulation of myofascial trigger points evokes segmental anti-nociceptive effects. J Rehabil Med. 2010;42(5):463-468.12 | Page

259. Srbely JZ, Dickey JP, Lee D, Lowerison M. Dry needle stimulation of myofascial trigger points evokes segmental anti-nociceptive effects. J Rehabil Med 2010;42(5):463–8.

260. Stanley, K. Thompson, A. Hynes, C. Brakebusch, and F. Quondamatteo, "NADPH oxidase complex-derived reactive International Scholarly Research Notices 13 oxygen species, the actin cytoskeleton, and Rho GTPases in cell migration," Antioxidants & Redox Signaling, vol. 20, no. 13, pp. 2026–2042, 2013.

261. Stellon A. Neurogenic pruritus: an unrecognised problem? A retrospective case series of treatment by acupuncture. Acupunct Med. Dec 2002;20(4):186-190.

262. Su JW, Lim CH, Chua YL. Bilateral pneumothoraces as a complication of acupuncture. Singapore Med J. 2007;48(1):e32–3.

263. Svensson P, Minoshima S, Beydoun A, Morrow TJ, Casey KL. Cerebral processing of acute skin and muscle pain in humans. J Neurophysiol. Jul 1997;78(1):450-460.

264. T. A. Garvey, M. R. Marks, and S. W. Wiesel, "A prospective, randomized, double-blind evaluation of trigger-point injection therapy for low-back pain," Spine, vol. 14, no. 9, pp. 962–964, 1989.

265. T. M. Cummings and A. R. White, "Needling therapies in the management of myofascial trigger point pain: a systematic review," Archives of Physical Medicine and Rehabilitation, vol. 82, no. 7, pp. 986–992, 2001.

266. T. S. Kuan, C. Z. Hong, J. T. Chen, S. M. Chen, and C. H. Chien, "The spinal cord connections of the myofascial trigger spots," European Journal of Pain, vol. 11, no. 6, pp. 624–634, 2007.

267. T. S. Kuan, J. T. Chen, S. M. Chen, C. H. Chien, and C. Z. Hong, "Effect of botulinum toxin on endplate noise in myofascial trigger spots of rabbit skeletal muscle," American Journal of Physical Medicine and Rehabilitation, vol. 81, no. 7, pp. 512–520, 2002.

268. Taspinar, U. B. Aslan, N. Sabir, and U. Cavlak, "Implementation of matrix rhythm therapy and conventional massage in young females and comparison of their acute effects on circulation,"Journal of Alternative and Complementary Medicine, vol. 19, no. 10, pp. 826–832, 2013.

269. Teachey WS. Otolaryngic myofascial pain syndromes. Curr Pain Headache Rep. Dec 2004;8(6):457-462.

270. Tekin L, Akarsu S, Durmus O, Cakar E, Dincer U, Kiralp MZ. The effect of dry needling in the treatment of myofascial pain syndrome: a randomized double-blinded placebo-controlled trial. Clin Rheumatol. Nov 9 2012.

271. This article is of great interest for it allows a simple, cheap, and noninvasive method for imaging myofascial trigger points. There is great scope for further study, especially in outcome studies correlating trigger points with clinical findings.

272. This study confirms the understanding of the segmental pattern of myofascial pain.

273. Travel & Simons Myofascial Pain and Dysfunction: The Trigger Point Manual; Vol. 1. The Upper Half of Body; 1999

274. Travell J G, Bigelow N H Referred somatic pain does not follow a simple 'segmental' pattern. Federation Proceedings 5: 106, 1946

275. Treaster D, Marras WS, Burr D, Sheedy JE, Hart D. Myofascial trigger point development from visual and postural stressors during computer work. J Electromyogr Kinesiol. Apr 2006;16(2):115- 124.

276. Tsai C-T, Hsieh L-F, Kuan T-S, Kao M-J, Chou L-W, Hong C-Z. Remote effects of dry needling on the irritability of the myofascial trigger point in the upper trapezius muscle. Am J Phys Med Rehabil. 2010;89(2):133-140.

277. Tsai CT, Hsieh LF, Kuan TS, Kao MJ, Chou LW, Hong CZ. Remote effects of dry needling on the irritability of the myofascial trigger point in the upper trapezius muscle. Am J Phys Med Rehabil 2010;89(2):133–40.

278. United States Department of Labor OSHA. Occupational Safety and Health Standards, Z, Toxic and Hazardous Substances, 1910.1030. Bloodborne pathogens. Washington, DC: United States Department of Labor, Occupational Safety & Health Administration.

279. Venancio Rde A, Alencar Jr FG, Zamperini C. Botulinum toxin, lidocaine, and dry-needling injections in patients with myofascial pain and headaches. Cranio. 2009;27(1):46–53.

280. W.H.McNulty, R.N.Gevirtz,D. R.Hubbard, andG.M. Berkoff, "Needle electromyographic evaluation of trigger point response to a psychological stressor," Psychophysiology, vol. 31, no. 3, pp. 313–316, 1994.

281. Wang C-F, Chen M, Lin M-T, Kuan T-S, Hong CZ. Teres minor tendinitis manifested with chronic myofascial pain syndrome in the scapular muscles; a case report. J Musculoskeletal Pain. 2006;14(1):39-43.

282. Weiner DK, Schmader KE. Postherpetic pain: more than sensory neuralgia? Pain Med. May-Jun 2006;7(3):243-249.

283. Weiss JM. Pelvic floor myofascial trigger points: manual therapy for interstitial cystitis and the urgency-frequency syndrome. J Urol. Dec 2001;166(6):2226-2231.

284. Whisler SL, Lang DM, Armstrong M, Vickers J, Qualls C, Feldman JS. Effects of myofascial release and other advanced myofascial therapies on children with cerebral palsy: six case reports. Explore. May-Jun 2012;8(3):199-205.

285. White A, Hayhoe S, Hart A, Ernst E. Adverse events following acupuncture: prospective survey of 32 000 consultations with doctors and physiotherapists. BMJ. 2001;323(7311):485–6.

286. White PF, Craig WF, Vakharia AS, Ghoname E, Ahmed HE, Hamza MA. Percutaneous neuromodulation therapy: does the location of electrical stimulation effect the acute analgesic response? Anesth Analg. Oct 2000;91(4):949-954.

287. Witt CM, Pach D, Brinkhaus B, et al. Safety of acupuncture: results of a prospective observational study with 229,230 patients and introduction of a medical information and consent form. Forsch Komplementmed. 2009;16(2):91–7.

288. Wittmann and C. M. Waterman-Storer, "Cell motility: can Rho GTPases and microtubules point the way?" Journal of Cell Science, vol. 114, part 21, pp. 3795–3803, 2001.

289. Wolfe, D. G. Simons, J. Fricton et al., "The fibromyalgia and myofascial pain syndromes: a preliminary study of tender points and trigger points in persons with fibromyalgia, myofascial pain syndrome and no disease," The Journal of Rheumatology, vol. 19, no. 6, pp. 944–951, 1992.

290. X. C. Santos, N. Anilkumar, M. Zhang, A. C. Brewer, and A. M. Shah, "Redox signaling in cardiac myocytes," Free Radical Biology and Medicine, vol. 50, no. 7, pp. 777–793, 2011.

291. Xu YM, Ge HY, Arendt-Nielsen L. Sustained nociceptive mechanical stimulation of latent myofascial trigger point induces central sensitization in healthy subjects. J Pain. 2010;11(12):1348-1355.

292. Y. L. Hsieh and C. Z. Hong, "Laser therapy for myofascial pain," Critical Reviews in Physical and Rehabilitation Medicine, vol. 22, no. 1–4, pp. 241–278, 2010

293. Y. L. Hsieh, L. W. Chou, Y. S. Joe, and C. Z. Hong, "Spinal cord mechanism involving the remote effects of dry needling on the irritability of myofascial trigger spots in rabbit skeletal muscle," Archives of Physical Medicine and Rehabilitation, vol. 92, no. 7, pp. 1098–1105, 2011.

294. Y. L. Hsieh, M. J. Kao, T. S. Kuan, S. M. Chen, J. T. Chen, and C. Z. Hong, "Dry needling to a key myofascial trigger point may reduce the irritability of satellite MTrPs," American Journal of Physical Medicine and Rehabilitation, vol. 86, no. 5, pp. 397–403, 2007.

295. Y. T. Huang, S. Y. Lin, C. A. Neoh, K. Y. Wang, Y. H. Jean, and H. Y. Shi, "Dry needling for myofascial pain: prognostic factors," Journal of Alternative and Complementary Medicine, vol. 17, no. 8, pp. 755–762, 2011. ·

296. Y.-C. Poh, S. Na, F. Chowdhury, M. Ouyang, Y. Wang, and N. Wang, "Rapid activation of Rac GTPase in living cells by force is independent of Src," PLoSONE, vol. 4, no. 11, Article IDe7886, 2009.

297. Yamashita H, Tsukayama H, Tanno Y, Nishijo K. Adverse events in acupuncture and moxibustion treatment: a six-year survey at a national clinic in Japan. J Altern Complement Med. 1999;5 (3):229–36.

298. Z. Hong and D. G. Simons, "Pathophysiologic and electrophysiologic mechanisms of myofascial trigger points," Archives of Physical Medicine and Rehabilitation, vol. 79, no. 7, pp. 863–872, 1998.

299. Z. Hong, "Research on myofascial pain syndrome," Critical Reviews in Physical and Rehabilitation Medicine, vol. 20, no. 4, pp. 343–366, 2008.

300. Z. Hong, "Specific sequential myofascial trigger point therapy in the treatment of a patient with myofascial pain syndrome associated with reflex sympathetic dystrophy," Australasian Chiropractic & Osteopathy, vol. 9, 7, no. 1, p. 11, 2000.